101 BEST ABS MOVES

by Jon Lipsey and Joel Snape

Art Editor Ian Ferguson
Managing Editor Chris Miller
Photography Glen Burrows
Model Tom Eastham
Cover Model Jay Conroy
Editorial Director Joe Warner

Publisher Steven O'Hara
Publishing Director Dan Savage
Marketing Manager Charlotte Park
Commercial Director Nigel Hole

Printed by William Gibbons and Sons, Wolverhampton

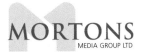

Published by Mortons Media Group Ltd,
Media Centre, Morton Way,
Horncastle, LN9 6JR
01507 529529

Contents

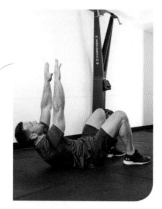

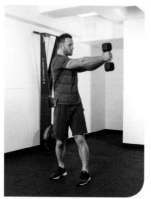

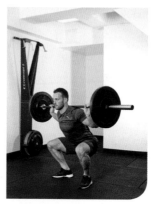

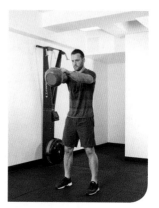

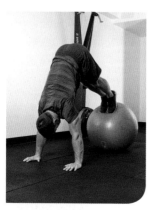

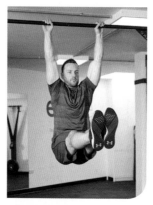

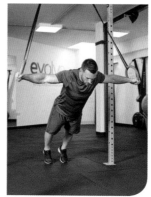

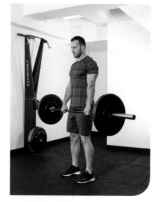

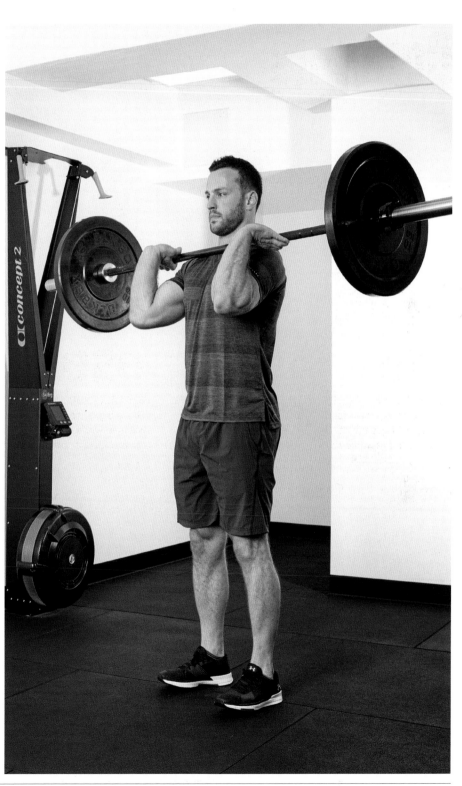

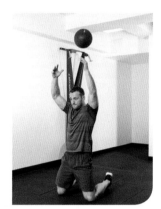
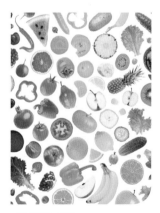

Your six-pack starts here

Get ready to reveal your abs by using exercises that work and a plan that gets results

Welcome to *101 Best Abs Moves*, your complete guide to building a rock-solid six-pack. In this book we've selected the most effective moves, using a range of training kit, that will help you hit your abs-sculpting goals.

The key to developing impressive abs is to work the abdominals, lower back and core from a variety of angles so that you get balanced muscle growth. Doing endless crunches won't cut it but doing a mixture of moves that target your upper, lower and side abs, as well as your deep-lying stabilising muscles, will have a positive effect.

To help you select the right moves for you, we've identified which section of the abs each exercise focuses on and we've also given each move a difficulty rating. Start with the easier exercises and increase the level of difficulty as you progress. The difficulty doesn't increase as you go through the secction, though – exercises are listed in alphabetical order to make them easier to find.

PLAN FOR SUCCESS

You can use this book in a couple of different ways. You can use it as inspiration for your abs workouts by selecting a couple of moves to add to the end of a standard training session. Or you can use the six-week training plan that starts on p128 to follow a structured approach to sculpting a six-pack.

And remember, while the activity of training your abs is done in the gym, some of the work has to be done in the kitchen, so follow our simple nutrition tips (p158) to ensure that you can reduce your body fat levels and show off your newly built muscle.

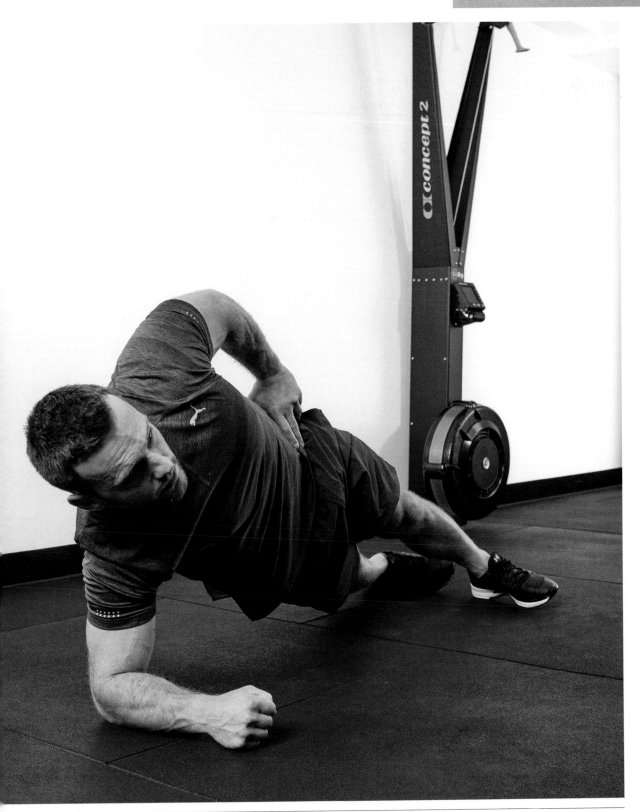

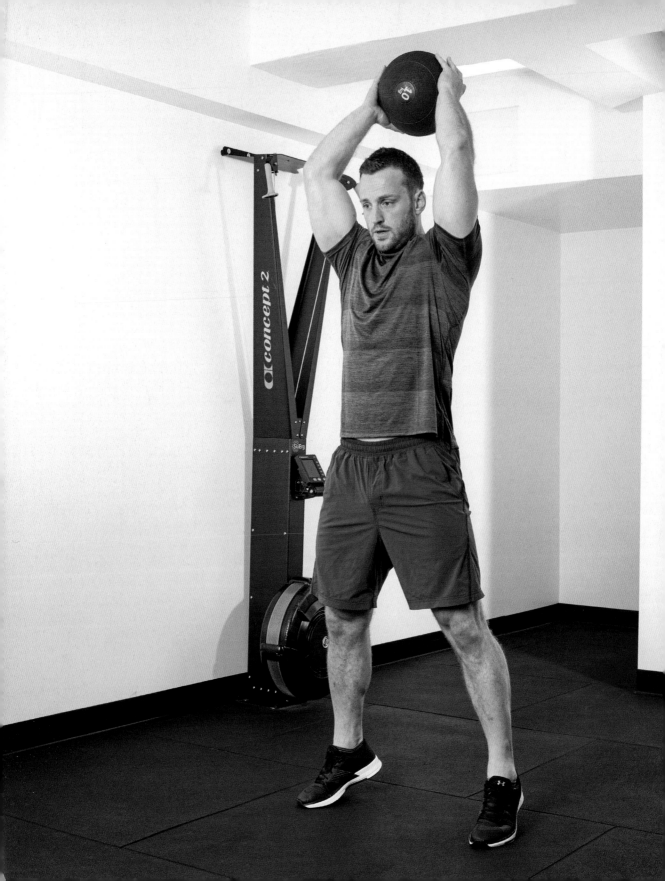

101 BEST ABS MOVES

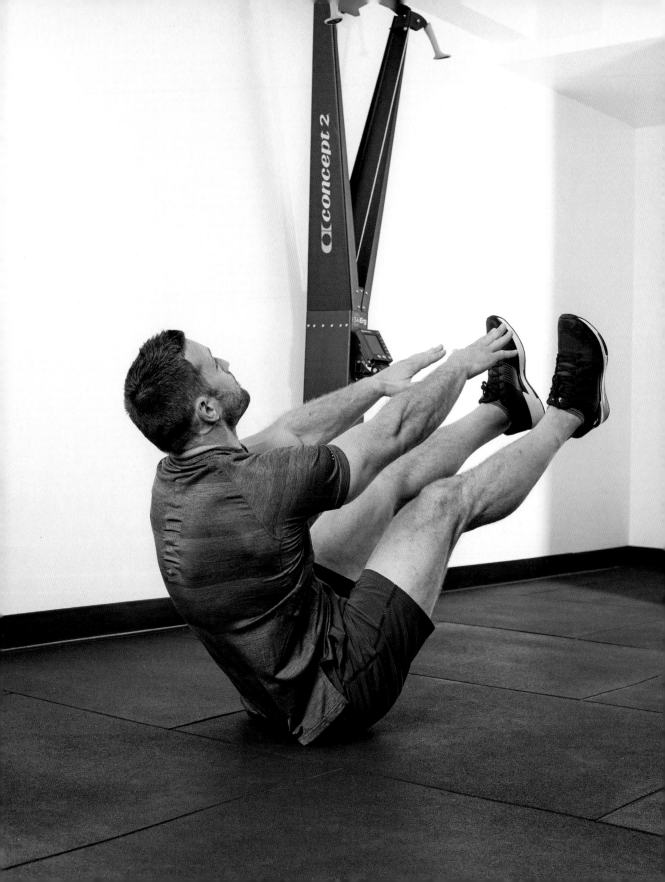

BODYWEIGHT EXERCISES

01 Bicycle

TARGET Upper, lower and side abs

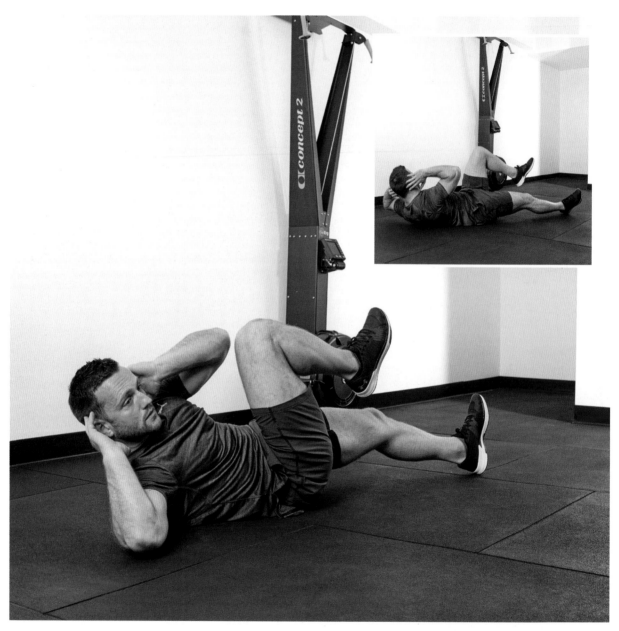

WHY This move's a three-in-one: keeping your legs elevated targets the lower abs, but the crunching and twisting motion also targets the upper abs and obliques, while helping with rotational strength.

HOW Lie on the floor with your fingertips by your head and feet slightly off the floor. Bring one knee up and move your opposite elbow towards it, then lower and repeat the move on the other side.

02 Crunch

TARGET Upper abs

DIFFICULTY RATING ⊙⊙⊙⊙⊙

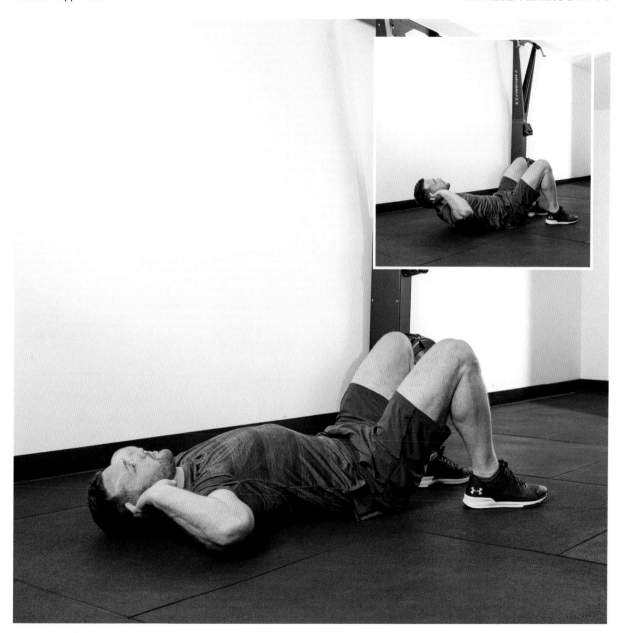

WHY By keeping things slower and more controlled than the traditional sit-up, the crunch targets the core rather than hip flexors, while minimising stress on your lower back. It's unfashionable, but still has a place in your routine.

HOW Lie flat on your back with knees bent and hands touching your temples. Contract your abs to raise your shoulders and curl your chest towards your knees. Pause at the top and squeeze your abs, then lower slowly to the start.

03 Crunch reach

TARGET Upper abs

DIFFICULTY RATING ⊙⊙⊙⊙⊙

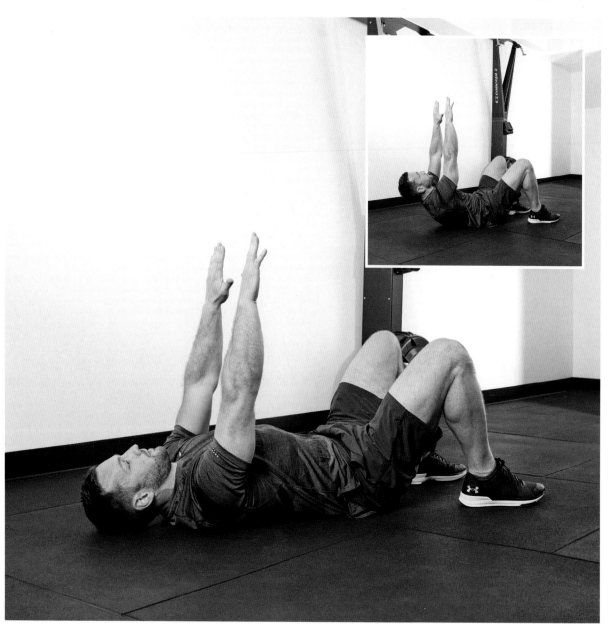

WHY This move forces you to keep the form strict, increasing the tension on your abs and the contraction at the top of the move for bigger gains.

HOW Lie on the floor with your knees bent and your arms raised vertically. Lift your upper back off the floor, still reaching straight upwards, pause and then lower.

04 Decline plank

TARGET Abs and core

DIFFICULTY RATING ●●●○○

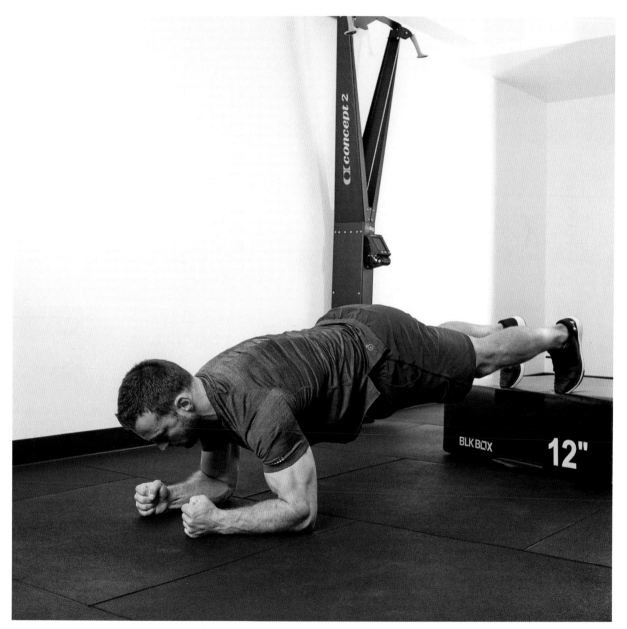

WHY By elevating your feet you'll put more training stress on your shoulders and change the angle your abs are working at, making the plank (see p22) tougher. For an even tougher variation, do it with your feet in suspension trainer straps.

HOW Get into a plank position with your forearms on the floor and feet on a box, bench or sofa, keeping your body completely straight. To make the move even tougher, move your elbows forwards and closer together.

05 Dish hold

TARGET Abs and core

DIFFICULTY RATING ●●●●●

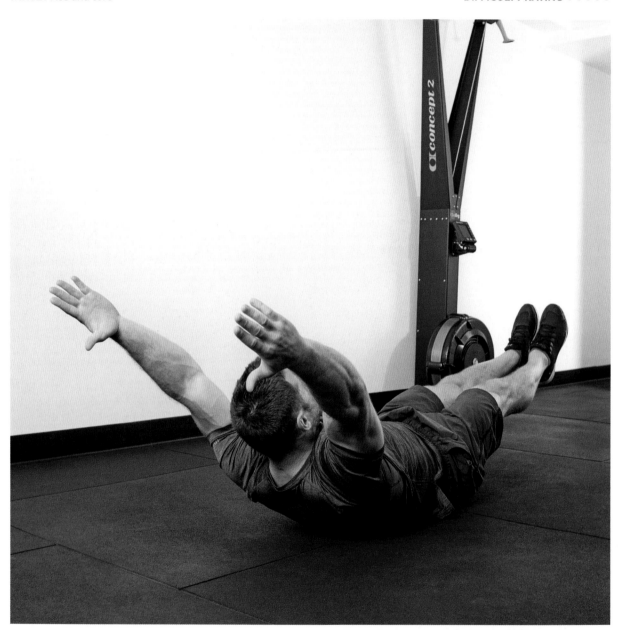

WHY It works your all abs muscles, including the deep-lying stability muscles, as well as strengthening your lower back.

HOW Lie on your back with your arms and legs fully extended. Contract your abs and raise your hands and feet off the floor. Maintain this tension on your core for 20 seconds without letting your hands or feet touch the floor.

06 Heel touch

TARGET Side abs

DIFFICULTY RATING ⊙ ⊙ ⊙ ⊙ ⊙

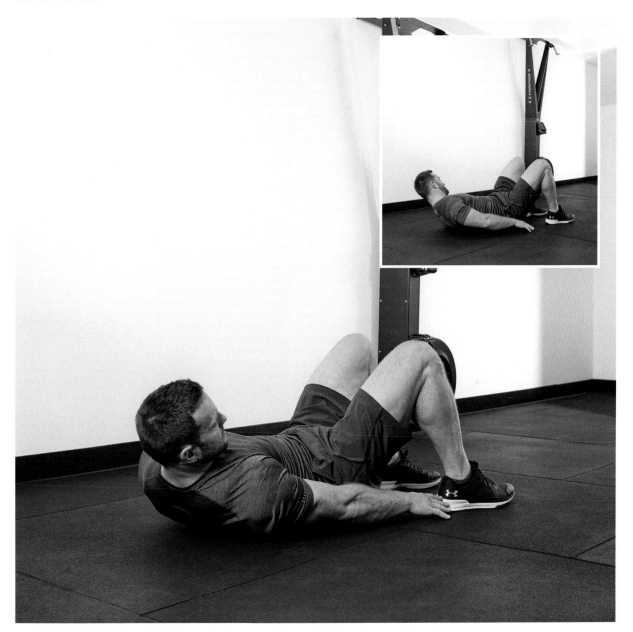

WHY Far harder than it looks, this move works your upper abs and obliques.

HOW Lie with your upper back off the ground, knees bent and feet flat. Crunch and reach forwards with one straight arm to touch your ankle, then go back to the start and repeat on the other side. Keep your upper back raised throughout.

07 Kick-out

TARGET Side abs

DIFFICULTY RATING ⦾⦾⦾⦾⦿

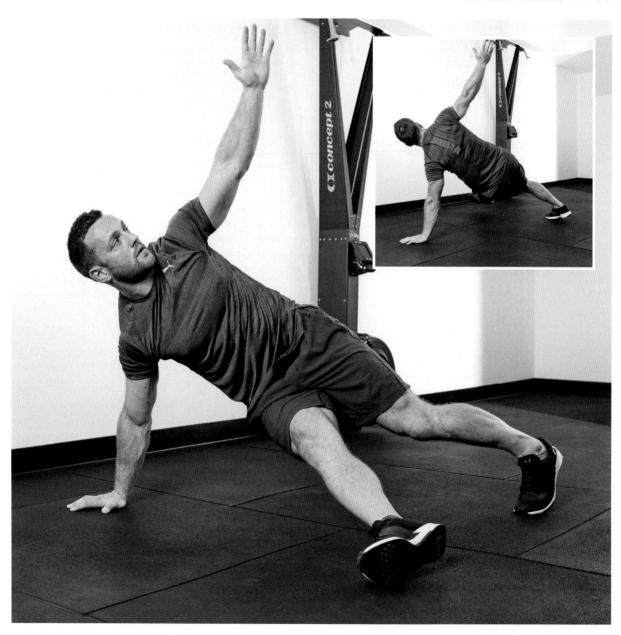

WHY A challenging but rewarding move that works your chest and shoulders as well as your abs.

HOW Perform a press-up then, as you return to the top, raise one arm and kick your other leg through under your body. Return to the start and repeat, kicking through to the other side. Engage your abs throughout.

08 Leg raise

TARGET Lower abs

DIFFICULTY RATING ⦿⦿⦾⦾⦾

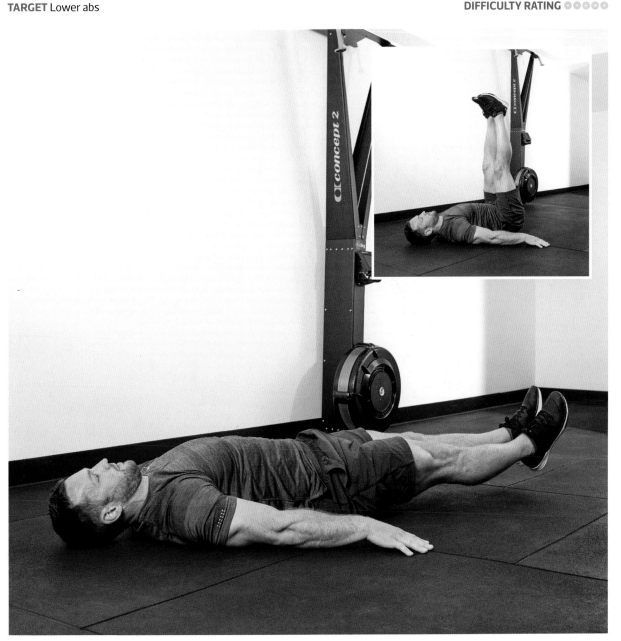

WHY One of the few bodyweight moves that targets the lower abs, the leg raise also strengthens the lower back, preventing injury.

HOW Lie on your back with your legs straight and heels slightly off the floor. Bring your legs up to a vertical position, then lower them slowly until they're just off the floor again.

09 Mountain climber

TARGET Upper, lower and side abs

DIFFICULTY RATING ⊙⊙⊙⊙⊙

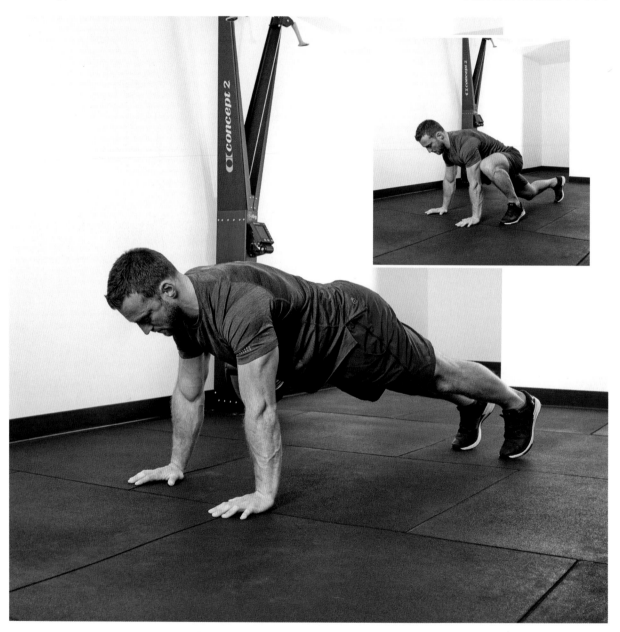

WHY This move can be done for speed and fat loss with high reps and short toe-touches on the floor. But bringing your knee up towards your chest works your abs too.

HOW Start in a position similar to a sprinter on the starting blocks. Bring one knee forwards, then back to the start. Repeat with the other leg. Keep the movement slow and controlled.

10 Pike crunch

TARGET Upper and lower abs

DIFFICULTY RATING ○○○○○

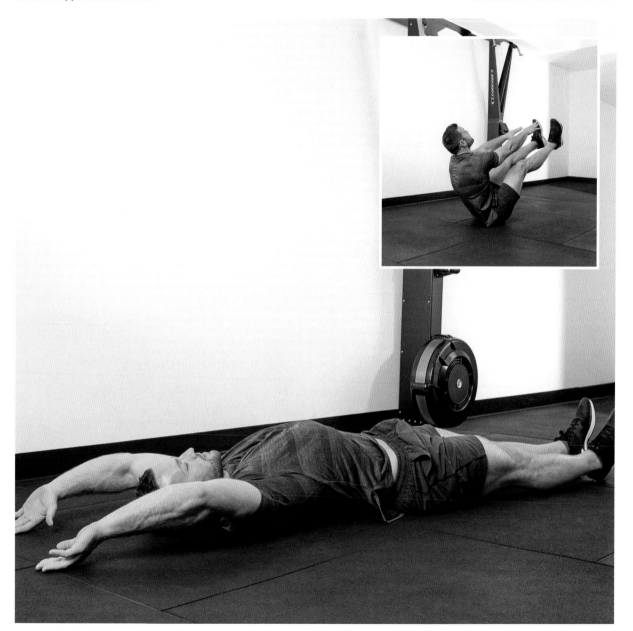

WHY Though most abs moves are prone to a bit of cheating, it's hard to do that with the pike crunch – it's pretty much self-correcting. Do it with your arms and body straight, and it ensures all the focus is on your abs.

HOW Lie on your back with your arms raised above your head. Engage your chest and crunch up as you bring your knees in towards you. Pause at the top, then lower under control.

11 Plank

TARGET Abs and core

DIFFICULTY RATING ●●○○○

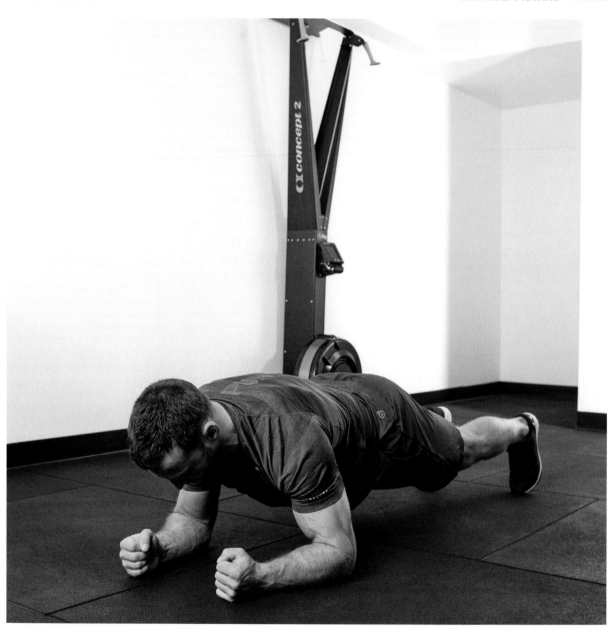

WHY The plank teaches your core muscles to maintain tension while improving your stability and posture and working your abs. Make sure you can hold this move for two minutes before doing more advanced abs training.

HOW Get into a press-up position but with your elbows and forearms on the floor and feet close together, keeping your body completely straight. Hold the position. To make the move tougher, move your elbows forwards and together.

12 Plank with leg raise

TARGET Abs and core

DIFFICULTY RATING ⊙⊙⊙⊙⊙

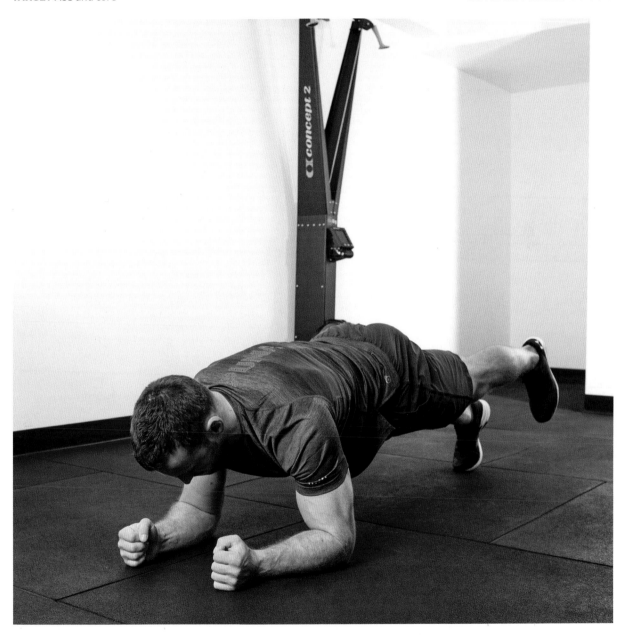

WHY Raising your legs alternately will force your entire core to remain activated for the full period of the hold.

HOW Start in the plank position. Raise one foot as high as you can, keeping your leg straight. Lower it, then raise your other leg. Keep each rep smooth and controlled, and hold your foot in the top position briefly to work the abs harder.

13 Plank touch

TARGET Abs and core

DIFFICULTY RATING ◐◐◐○○

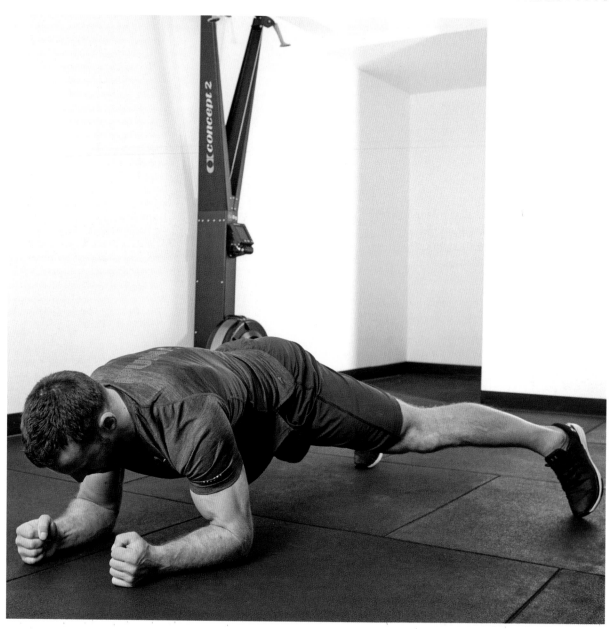

WHY Moving your leg off the floor creates a higher level of instability, which makes the move more difficult and also challenges your abs in a different way.

HOW Get into the plank position then raise one leg and place it 30–40cm away from the start position. Return to the start and perform the same movement on the other side.

14 Reverse crunch

TARGET Lower abs

DIFFICULTY RATING ⊙⊙⊙⊙⊙

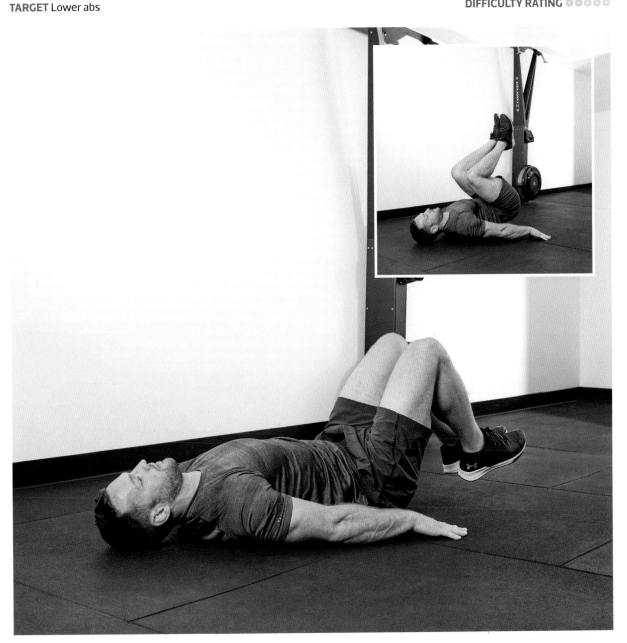

WHY The reverse crunch is one of the few moves you can do without a pull-up bar to target the lower abs. Use it alongside the standard crunch for an abs double whammy.

HOW Lie flat on your back with knees bent and arms flat against the floor. Contract your lower abs to draw your knees in towards your chest. Pause at the top of the move and squeeze your abs, then return to the start.

15 Rolling plank

TARGET Abs and core

DIFFICULTY RATING ○○○○○

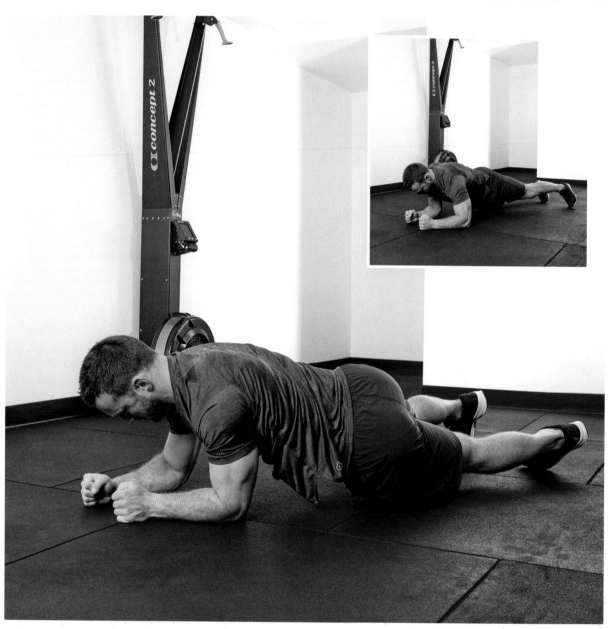

WHY A tough variation on the classic plank that places more emphasis on your obliques.

HOW Start in the plank position. Roll to one side so that your hip touches the floor, then roll back to repeat this on the other side. Continue alternating, keeping the movement slow and controlled.

16 Russian twist

TARGET Side abs

DIFFICULTY RATING ●●●●●

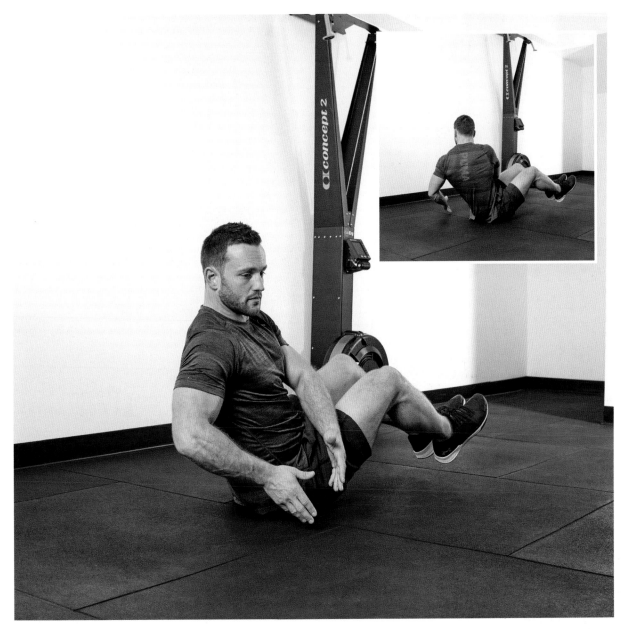

WHY This rotational move works your obliques and entire core to give you a strong foundation for all sports.

HOW Sit with your body at around 45° to the floor, with your knees bent and back straight. Raise your arms slightly and twist your torso to one side, maintaining the angle of your upper body to the floor. Then twist to the other side.

17 Side crunch

TARGET Side abs

DIFFICULTY RATING ⊙⊙⊙⊙⊙

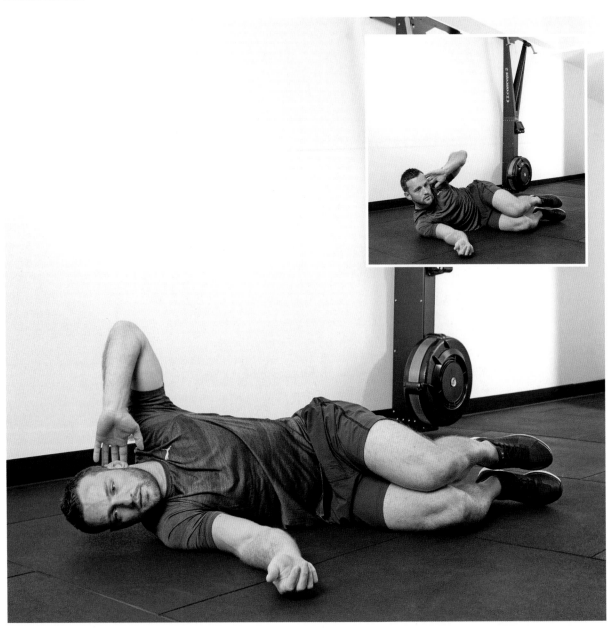

WHY This move works your abs and obliques in one motion, while building the twisting strength that helps in numerous sports.

HOW Lie on the floor on your side with your knees bent. With one hand by the side of your head, flex your abs and raise your shoulders off the floor. Pause, then lower.

18 Side plank

TARGET Abs and core

DIFFICULTY RATING ●●●●●

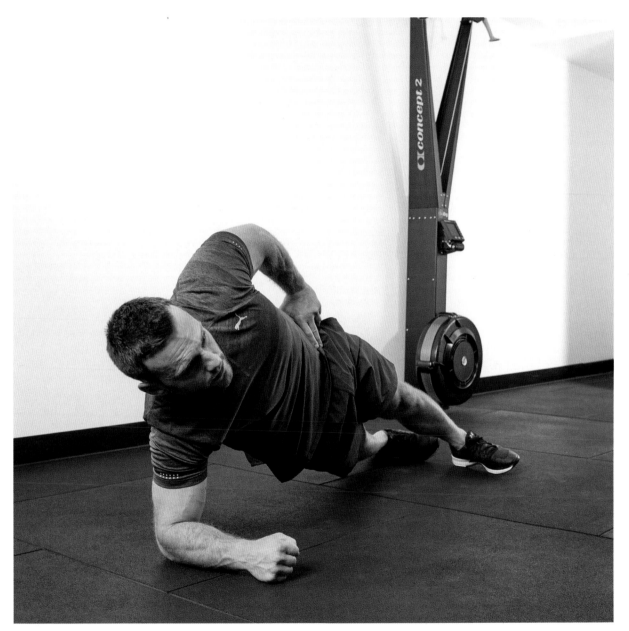

WHY Shifting onto one side hits your obliques harder than the traditional plank. Put them together into a superset – 30 seconds of plank, 30 seconds on one side, 30 more seconds of plank, and a final 30 seconds on the other side.

HOW Rest on one forearm with your feet "stacked" one on top of the other – or both on the floor, one behind the other (known as "staggered") if this is too hard. Keep your body in a straight line – once you start to sag, the set's over.

19 Side plank crunch

TARGET Abs and core

DIFFICULTY RATING ●●●○○

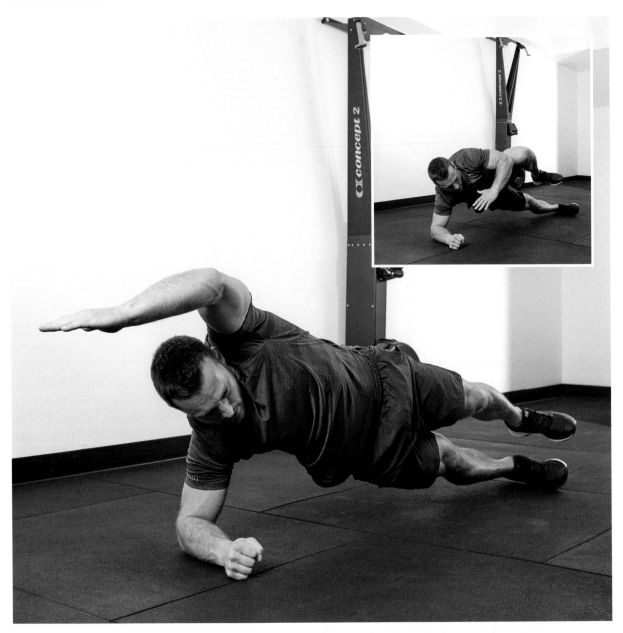

WHY Another move that works your obliques, while the crunch movement recruits the small stabilising muscles that keep you balanced

HOW Start in a side plank position. Hold your top arm straight out next to your head with your top leg raised. Contract your abs to bring your elbow and knee together, then straighten both back out. Swap sides for the second set.

20 Side plank raise

TARGET Abs and core

DIFFICULTY RATING ●●●○○

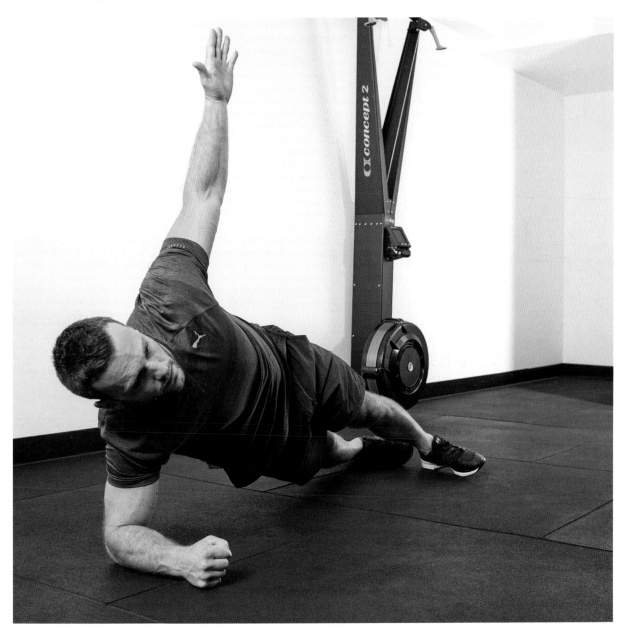

WHY This variation of the side plank – popular with yogis – demands more coordination and balance than the standard position, and it's more challenging.

HOW Lie in a side plank position on one hand, feet stacked. Raise your arm and hold. Repeat on the other side.

21 Spider-Man press-up

TARGET Abs and core

DIFFICULTY RATING ○○○○○

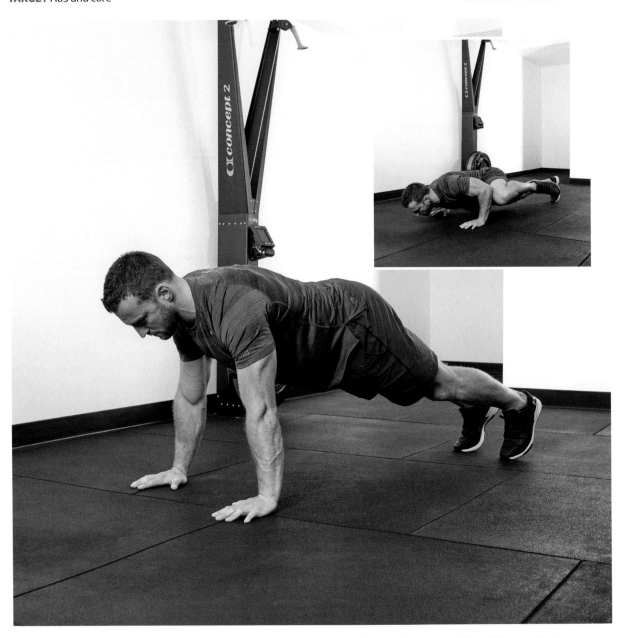

WHY Taking one foot off the floor forces your stabiliser muscles to work overtime, as well as activating your core to stabilise your torso. For best results, keep the reps slow and controlled, and your body parallel to the floor throughout.

HOW Perform a press-up position, lifting one foot off the floor and raise the knee to your elbow as you lower. Press back up, placing your foot back on the floor. Repeat on the other side.

22 Squat thrust

TARGET Upper and lower abs

DIFFICULTY RATING ○ ○ ○ ○ ○

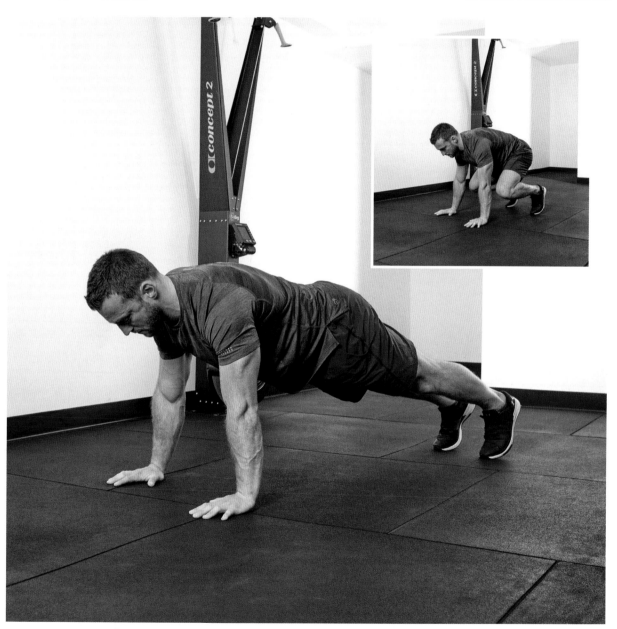

WHY The movement of bringing your feet from the press-up position to below your chest recruits the abs. The move also trains your ability to move explosively and decelerate.

HOW Get into a press-up position, then jump both feet forwards simultaneously so that they are below your chest, then jump your feet back.

23 T-raise

TARGET Abs and core

DIFFICULTY RATING ⦾⦾⦾⦿⦿

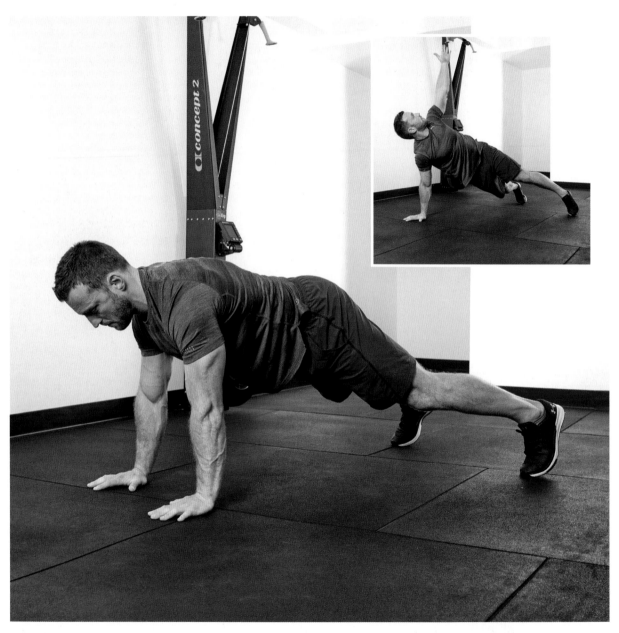

WHY Most people devote the majority of the time that they spend training their abs to movements that work in one plane. This exercise trains your midsection in the often neglected rotational plane.

HOW Start in the top of a press-up position, then rotate to open up your body and raise one arm until it is vertical. Then return to the start.

24 V–sit

TARGET Upper and lower abs

DIFFICULTY RATING ○○○○○

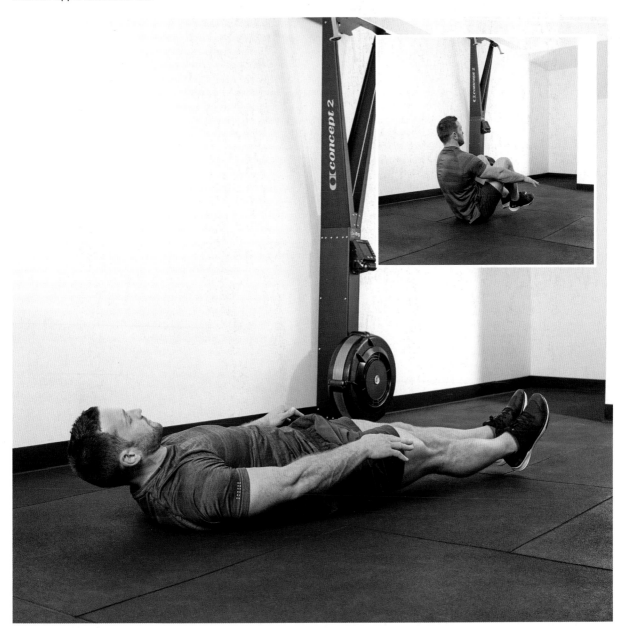

WHY Most people do this move explosively, but if you can do it slowly and under control, it's a sign that you've built serious abs strength. Still jerking your way through the movement? Regress to the pike crunch and work your way up.

HOW Lie on your back with your arms and legs straight. Bending your knees, raise your legs and upper body, stretching your arms past your shins. Hold this position for a moment, then go back to the start position.

25 Walk-out

TARGET Abs and core

DIFFICULTY RATING ○○○○○

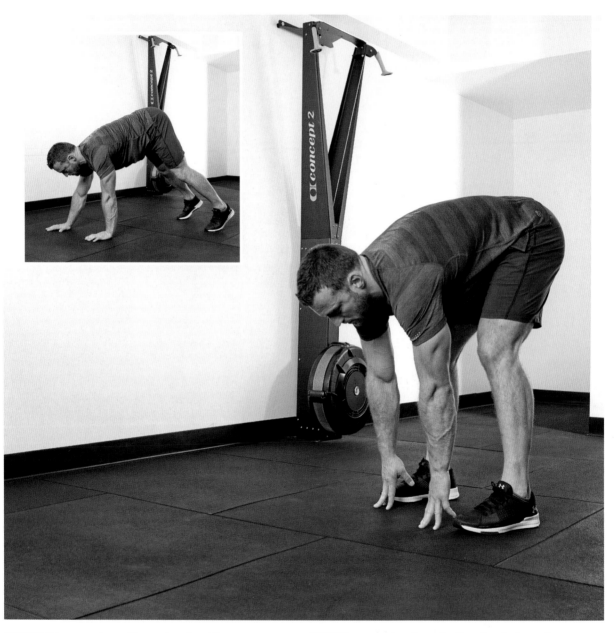

WHY Walking exercises with your hands on the floor get your body moving in a way many people neglect. This exercise allows you to move in a fluid way with a constantly adjusting core challenge.

HOW Place your hands on the floor just in front of your feet, then gradually 'walk' your hands forwards until you're in the top of a press-up position. Then walk your feet forwards gradually to return to the start.

26 Windscreen wiper

TARGET Side abs

DIFFICULTY RATING ○○○○○

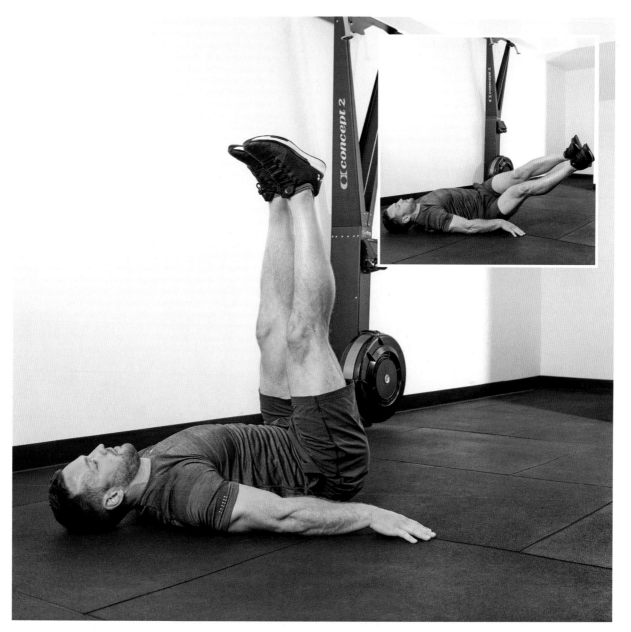

WHY This is a demanding move that tests your rotational strength because you have to control the movement of your legs, which increases in difficulty the further they lower.

HOW Lie on your back with your legs straight and raised. Twist to lower your feet to one side, then return to the start position and lower them on the other side.

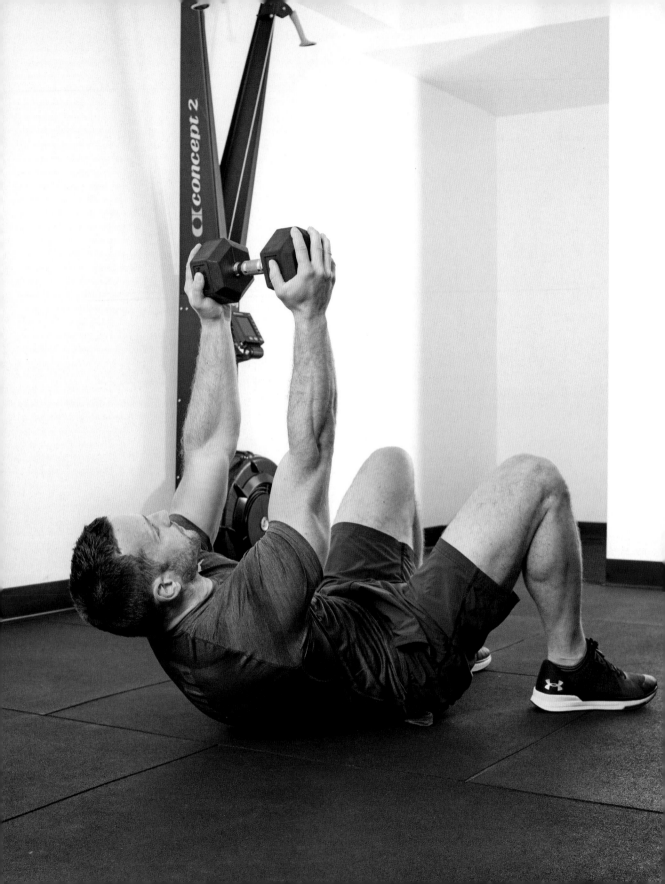

DUMBBELL EXERCISES

27 Crunch

TARGET Upper abs

DIFFICULTY RATING ●●○○○

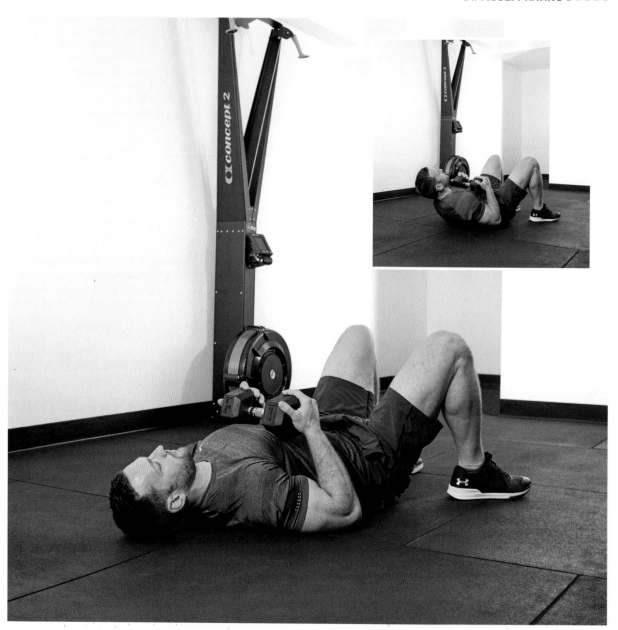

WHY In lab testing, weighted crunches activate the abs more than almost any other isolation move. Using a dumbbell (or weight plate) for slow, controlled reps is a great way to work your whole core.

HOW Lie flat on your back with knees bent and a dumbbell held at chest level. Contract your abs to raise your shoulders and curl your chest towards your knees. Pause at the top and squeeze your abs, then lower slowly back to the start.

28 Crunch reach

TARGET Upper abs

DIFFICULTY RATING ●●●○○

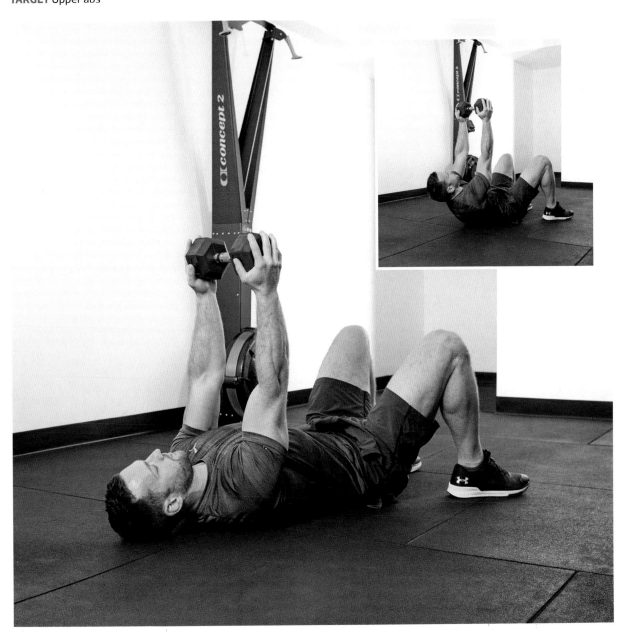

WHY Leading with the dumbbell discourages you from jerking, ensuring that the focus stays on your abs while safeguarding your lower back.

HOW Lie flat on your back with your knees bent and a dumbbell held above your chest with arms straight. Crunch up, pause at the top of the movement, then lower back to the start.

29 Halo

TARGET Abs and core

DIFFICULTY RATING ⊙⊕⊕⊕⊕

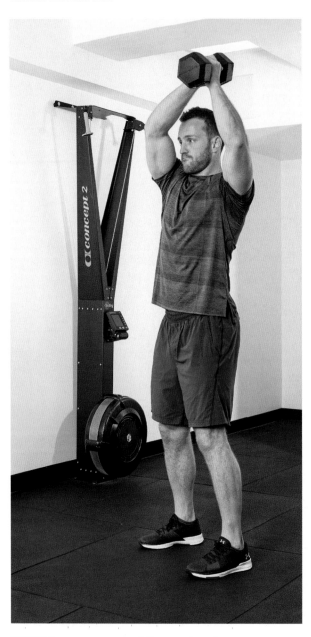
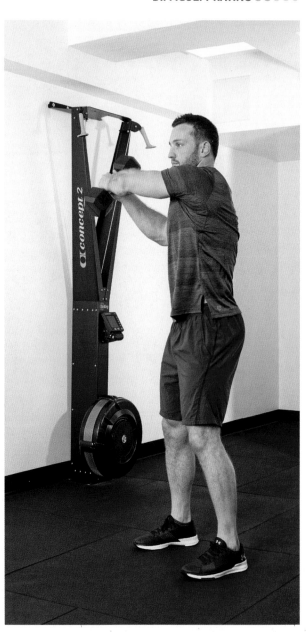

WHY This move engages all the muscles of your core and, because you're doing it from a standing position, teaches them to fire in practical situations.

HOW Holding a dumbbell in both hands, move it around your head, engaging your core as you circle it around. After one complete circle, reverse directions.

30 Overhead carry

TARGET Abs and core

DIFFICULTY RATING ●●●●●

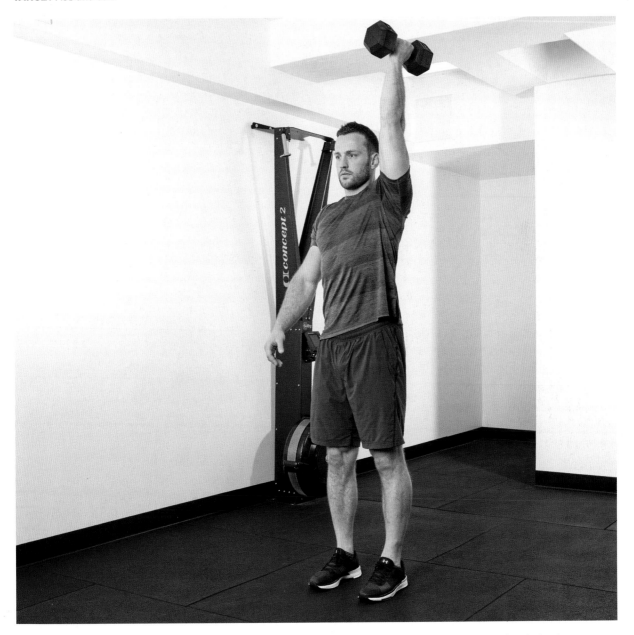

WHY Any carrying move is good for your abs and core but a unilateral one – where you're only carrying a weight in one hand – is best because your body has to resist the force dragging it out of alignment.

HOW Holding a dumbbell above your head, simply walk around for a set period of time. Then swap hands and do the same on the other side. Start with a light weight and increase the load as you get stronger.

31 Press-up renegade row

TARGET Abs and core

DIFFICULTY RATING ●●●○○

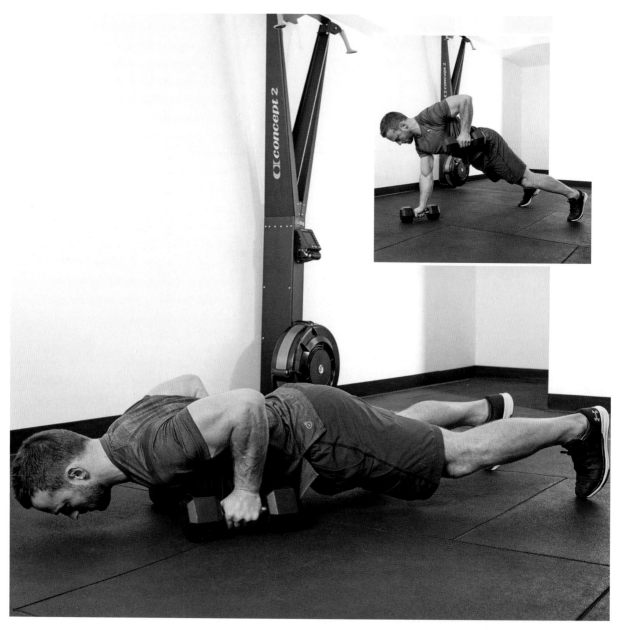

WHY Adding a press-up to the renegade row (see opposite) engages your chest – especially if you use the extra height to descend further into the move. It's pulling and pushing in one exercise, making this a great bang-for-your-buck move.

HOW Start in a press-up position holding a pair of dumbbells. Do a press-up. At the top of the move, row one dumbbell up (so that your thumb touches your armpit) and down, then the other. Try to stay parallel to the floor – don't twist.

32 Renegade row

TARGET Abs and core

DIFFICULTY RATING ●●●○○

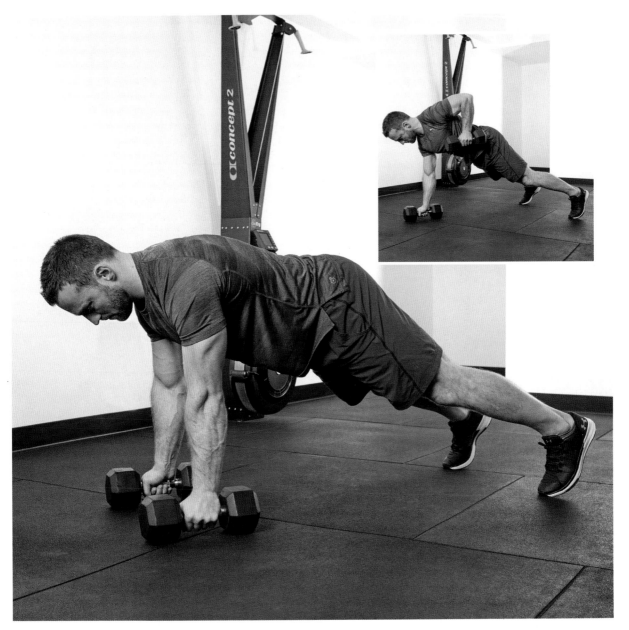

WHY This move works your back muscles while challenging your stabilisers to keep you level. Think of it as a brutal version of the plank. It's even tougher on rounded dumbbells.

HOW Start in a press-up position holding a pair of dumbbells. Row one dumbbell up (so that your thumb touches your armpit) and down, then the other. Try to stay parallel to the floor – don't twist.

33 Russian twist

TARGET Side abs

DIFFICULTY RATING ●●○○○

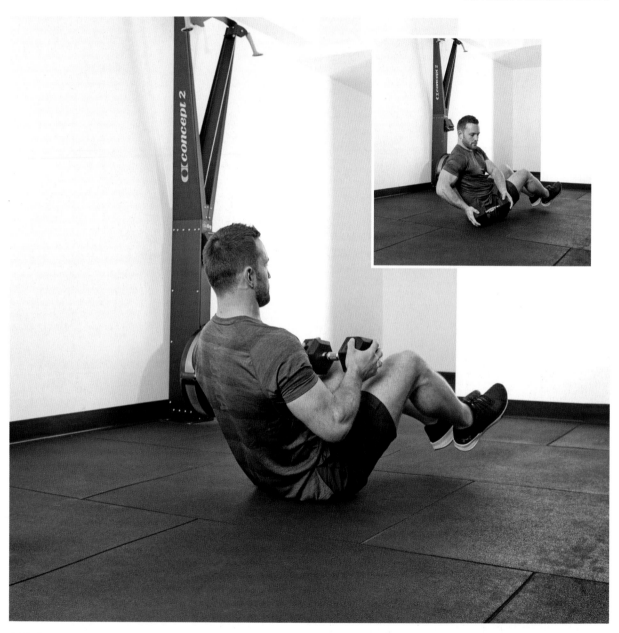

WHY Training with rotational moves is vital for sports performance and a well-rounded physique, and this is one of the safest ways to do it effectively.

HOW Sit with your body at around 45° to the floor, with your knees bent and back straight, holding a dumbbell in two hands. Twist your torso to one side, maintaining the angle of your upper body to the floor. Then twist to the other side.

34 Side bend

TARGET Side abs

DIFFICULTY RATING ○○○○○

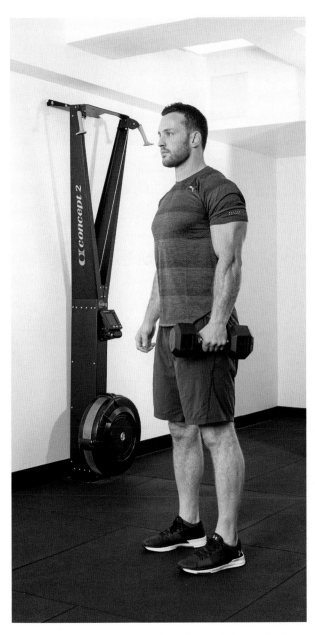
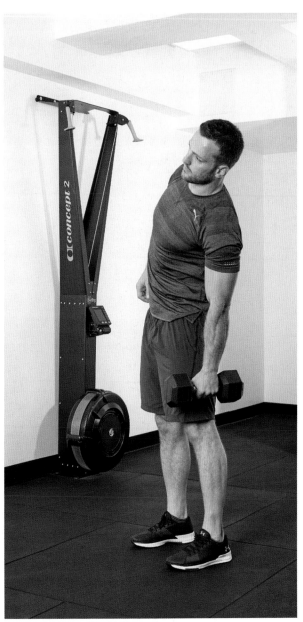

WHY As well as your obliques the side bend also works the muscles of your lower back, helping to protect your core.

HOW Hold a heavy dumbbell in one hand and bend your torso towards your weighted hand. Pause when you feel a stretch up your opposite side, then straighten up without leaning forwards or backwards.

35 Standing Russian twist

TARGET Side abs

DIFFICULTY RATING ●●●○○

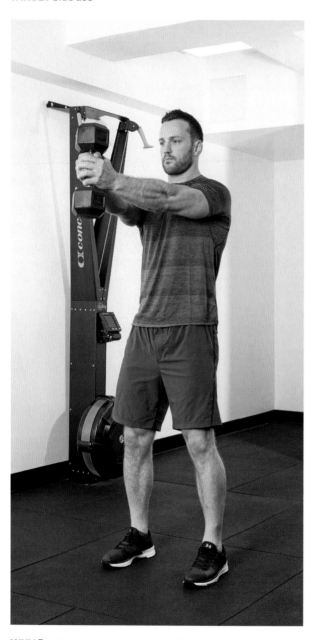
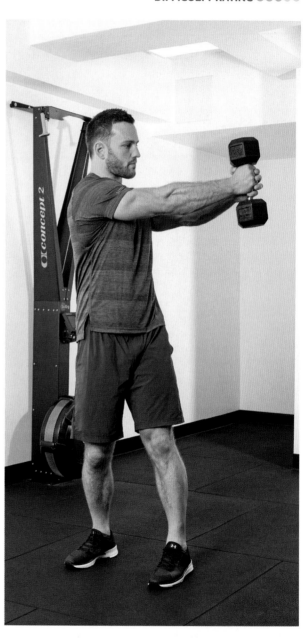

WHY Russian twists are usually performed while sitting on the floor (see p46). Doing it standing up changes the challenge because you have to resist the weight pulling you forwards.

HOW Stand up straight with your core braced and hold a dumbbell at chest height in front of you with your arms straight. Rotate your torso to move the weight to one side. Come back to the centre and repeat on the other side.

36 Woodchop

TARGET Side abs

DIFFICULTY RATING ⊕⊕⊙⊙⊙

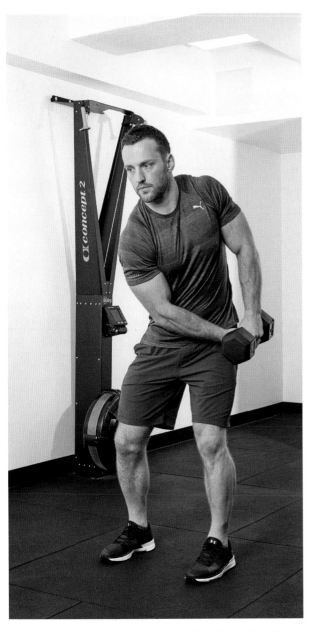
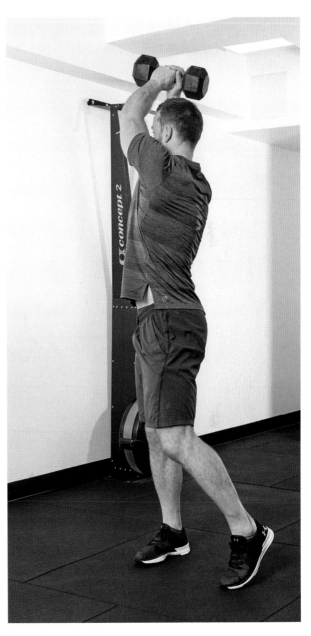

WHY Most abs moves work in the simpler planes of motion, such as the crunch, which works in the frontal plane. This move works in the rotational plane, which makes it functional and useful for everyday and sporting movements.

HOW Hold a dumbbell in both hands just outside your hip, with your torso upright and your knees bent slightly. Twist and move the weight up and across your body, straightening up as you go.

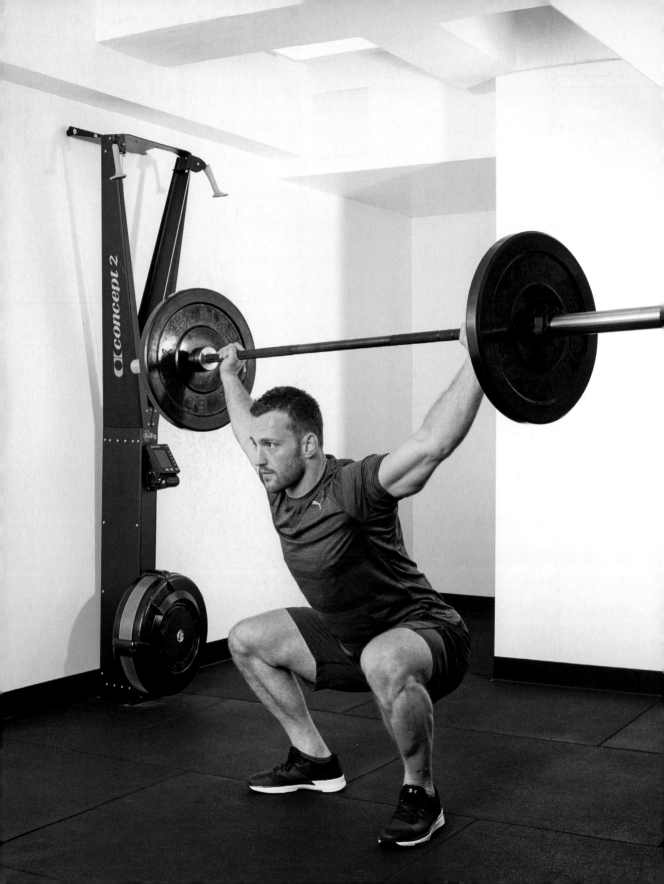

BARBELL EXERCISES

37 Bench press

TARGET Chest, triceps, abs

DIFFICULTY RATING ●●●○○

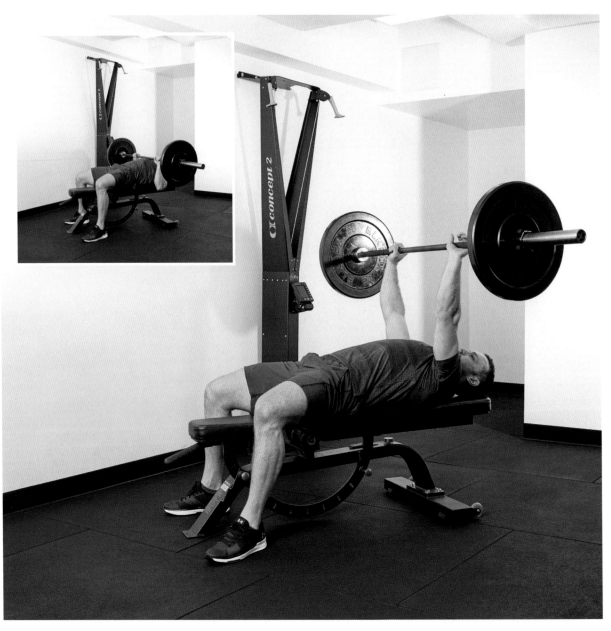

WHY It's a classic for a reason: a properly executed bench press (your feet should be pressing into the floor) will tax your whole body and allow you to use heavy weights to maximise upper-body development.

HOW Take a grip slightly wider than shoulder width and squeeze your lats together. Lower the bar to your chest, aiming to brush your T-shirt without bouncing. Press up powerfully, pause at the top, then do your next rep.

38 Bent-over row

TARGET Back, biceps and abs

DIFFICULTY RATING ●●●○○

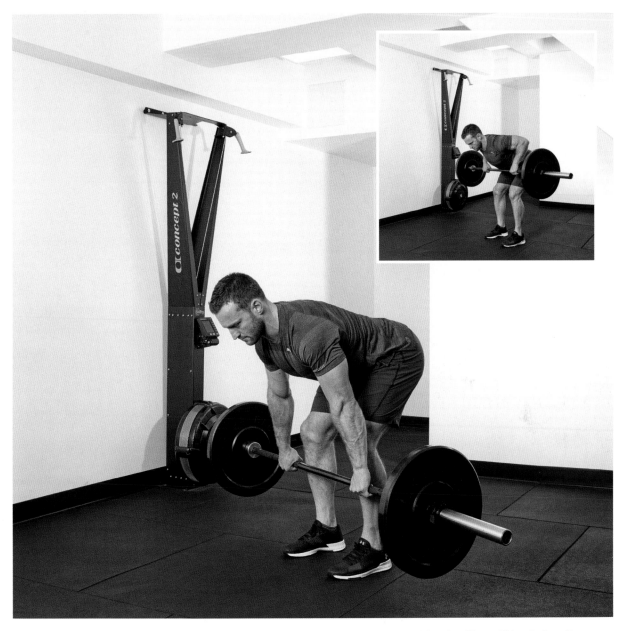

WHY It's the best back-builder bar none – but it'll also even out your pressing and give you a stable base for pushing-based moves. For a variation, try the Pendlay row, where each rep starts on the floor.

HOW Hold the bar with a shoulder-width grip, bending your knees slightly. Bend at the hips, then pull the bar up to your sternum and then lower under control. If you're moving your upper body to shift the bar, the weight's too heavy.

39 Deadlift

TARGET Whole body

DIFFICULTY RATING ⦿⦿⦿⦿○

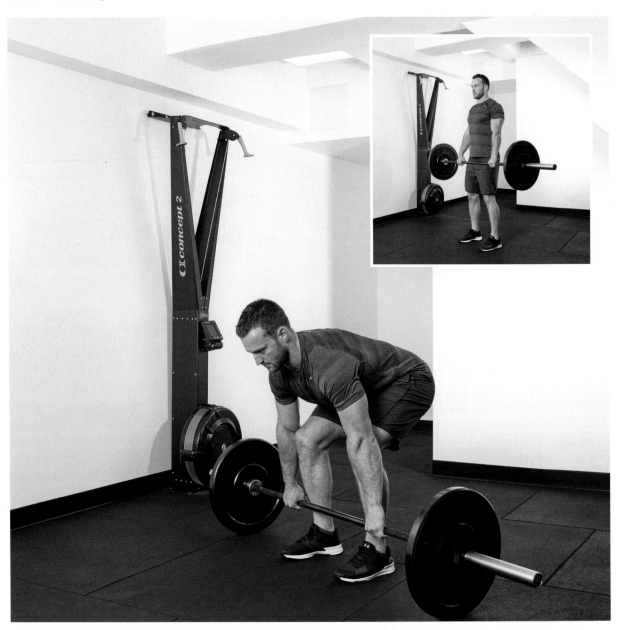

WHY It's the best full-body move bar none: if this was all you did, you'd still build enviable arms and a core of steel. It'll flood your body with testosterone and growth hormone, and let you lift heavier than almost any other move.

HOW Standing with your feet shoulder-width apart, grasp the bar with your hands just outside your legs. Lift the bar by driving your hips forward, keeping a flat back. Lower the bar under control (it's OK to drop it on your final rep).

40 Glute bridge

TARGET Glutes, hamstrings and abs

DIFFICULTY RATING ●●●○○

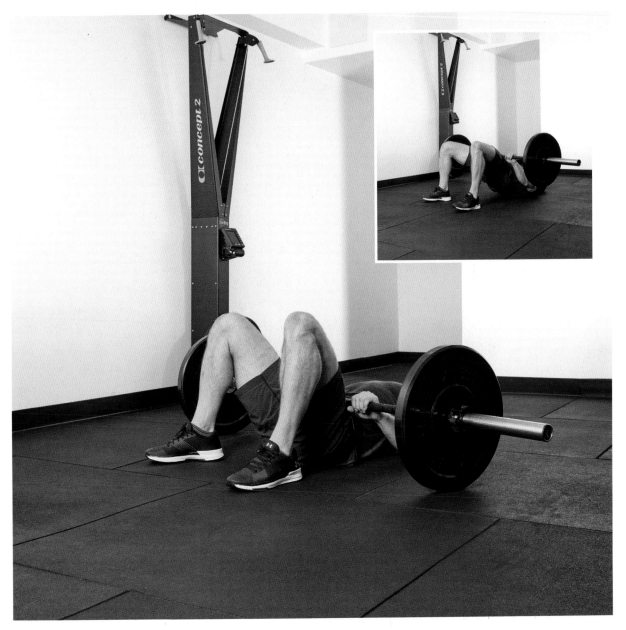

WHY This allows you to move big weights for increased glute activation – and it'll teach your glutes to 'fire' during squat variations.

HOW Position yourself with a barbell across your hips, your shoulders on the floor and your feet close to your glutes. Raise your hips until they're in line with your shoulders and knees. Hold for a second in the top position, then lower.

41 Good morning

TARGET Lower back and abs

DIFFICULTY RATING ●●●○○

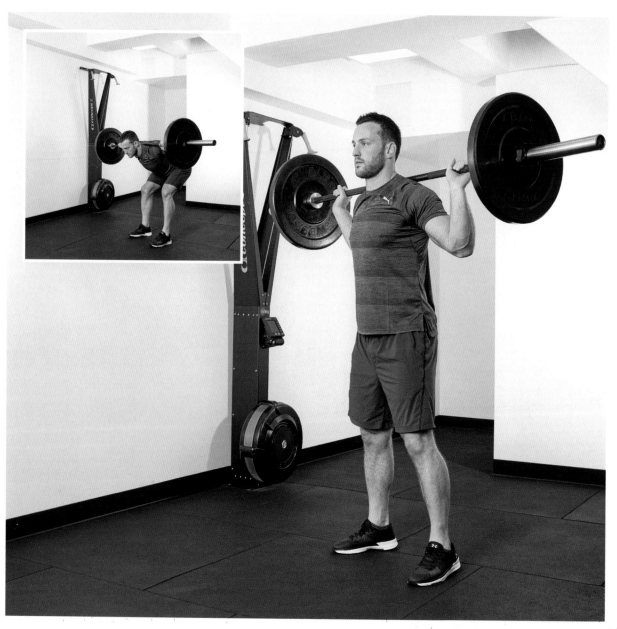

WHY This move will target the erector spinae muscles – the long back muscles that support the spine, which is important for executing abs moves safely. It will also help to improve your posture.

HOW **Place a barbell across your back and grip it with hands just wider than shoulder-width apart. Push your backside back to hinge at the hips until you feel a strong hamstring stretch, then straighten up.**

42 Kneeling roll-out

TARGET Abs and core

DIFFICULTY RATING ⦿⦿⦿⦿⦾

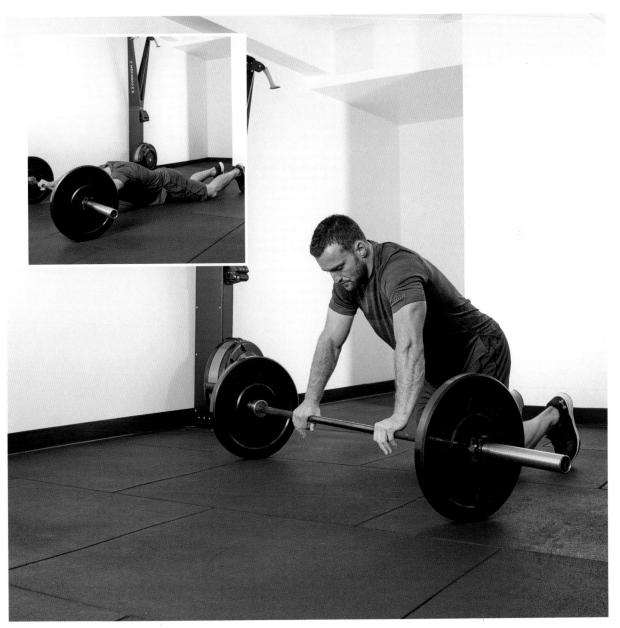

WHY This variation on the classic abs wheel roll-out is much tougher because of the added weight – although the bar does provide extra stability. Once you can do more than ten reps, increase the weight.

HOW Kneel holding a barbell with a shoulder-width grip. Slowly roll it away from you, keeping your core braced. Extend until your torso is parallel to the ground, then contract your abs to pull the bar back to the start.

43 Landmine

TARGET Abs and core

DIFFICULTY RATING ●●●●●

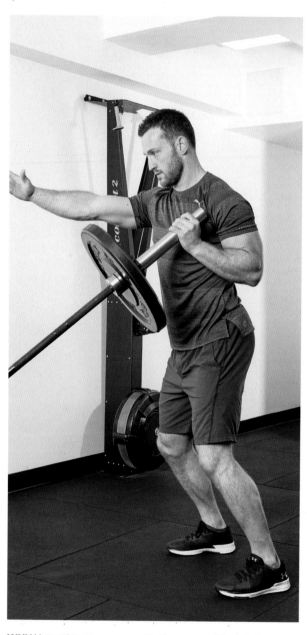
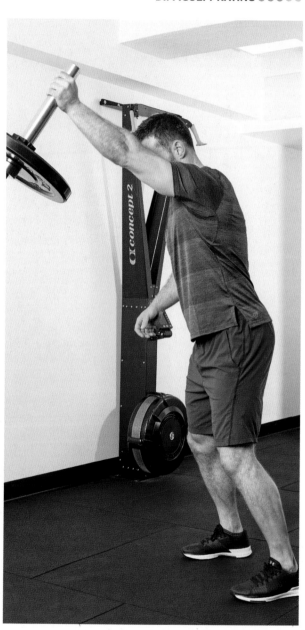

WHY Using this move – so called because of the bit of kit sometimes used to slot the barbell into – allows you to build strength from unusual angles, including the rotational power you'll need to throw a punch or a ball.

HOW Wedge a barbell into a weight plate or corner (or a landmine if your gym has one). Hold one end and twist on your back foot as if throwing a punch, then push the barbell away. Do all your reps on one side, then switch to the other.

44 Overhead press

TARGET Shoulders, triceps and abs

DIFFICULTY RATING ⊕⊕⊕⊕⊕

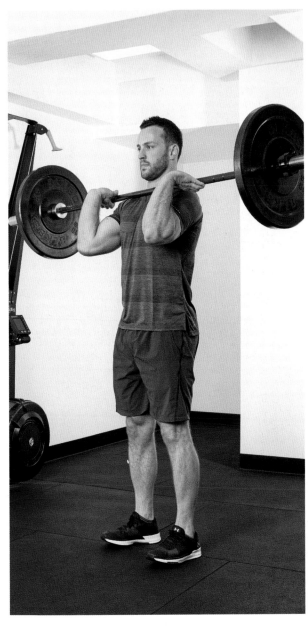

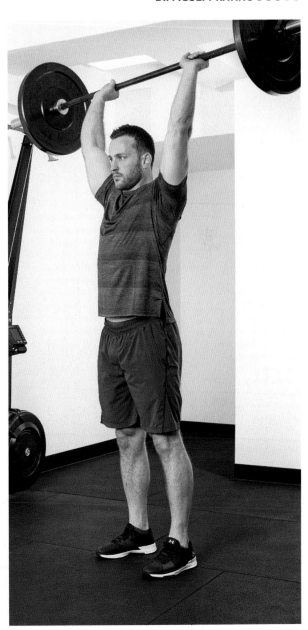

WHY The strict overhead press builds full-body muscle and coordination, bringing your abs into the equation to stabilise the weight you press overhead. The 'military' version – done with your feet together – is even tougher.

HOW Position a bar on your upper chest, gripping it with hands just wider than shoulder-width apart. Brace your abs, glutes and quads, then press the bar straight upwards. Pause at the top, then lower.

45 Overhead squat

TARGET Legs and abs

DIFFICULTY RATING ⊕⊕⊕⊕⊕

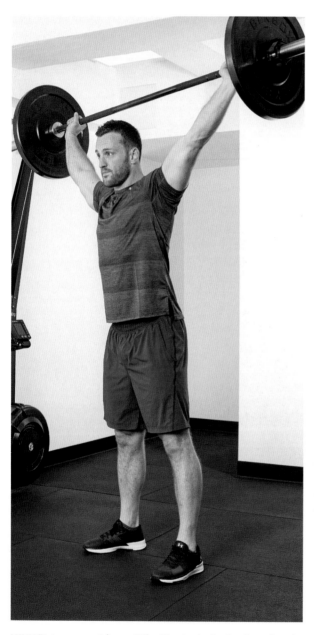

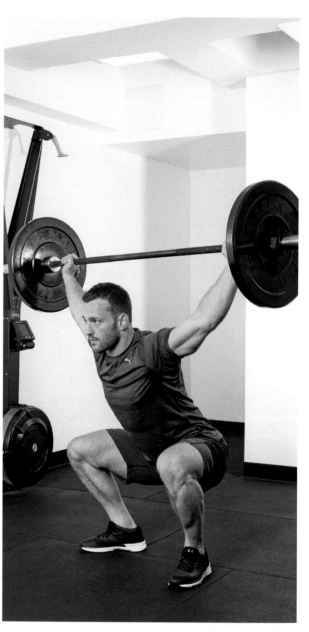

WHY Doing a sqaut (see p62) with a barbell raised overhead is a key test of shoulder, ankle and hip mobility. Start adding weight and you'll find it's a serious core builder that'll also prepare you for the rigours of Olympic weightlifting.

HOW Either press a bar overhead with your hands at double shoulder-width, or take it out of a rack. Think about pulling the bar apart to keep it stable as you lower into a squat, keeping your weight over your heels.

46 Roll-out

TARGET Abs and core

DIFFICULTY RATING ●●●●●

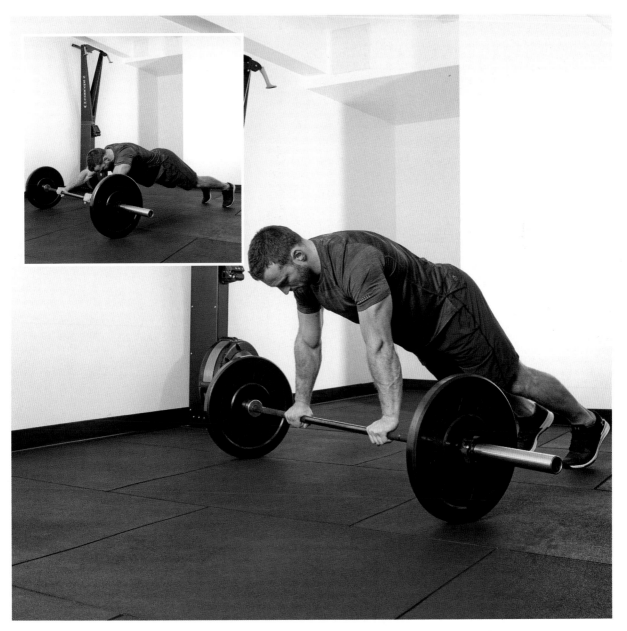

WHY Doing the roll-out on your feet rather than knees is extremely difficult, and you should attempt it only after you have mastered the kneeling version. But the reward is rock-solid abs and core control.

HOW Stand with your arms extended and slowly roll the bar away from you, keeping your core braced. Extend until your torso is parallel to the ground, then contract your abs to pull the bar back towards you to return to the start.

47 Squat

TARGET Legs and abs

DIFFICULTY RATING ●●●○○

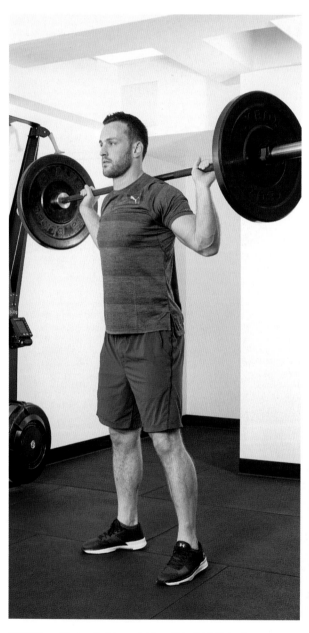

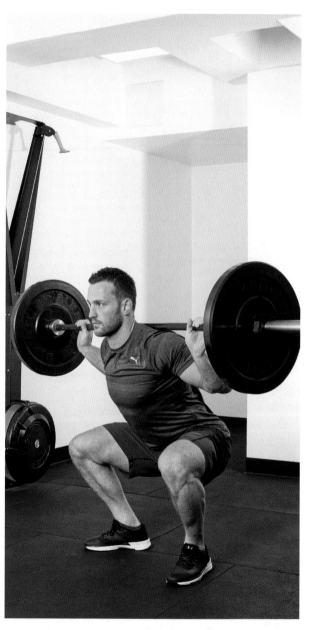

WHY Squatting with big weights will build full-body muscle thanks to the huge growth hormone hit it prompts. It works not just your core but also your legs, back and everything else below the bar.

HOW Hold the bar on your upper back and stand with feet shoulder-width apart, toes pointing out slightly. Lower as if you're aiming for a chair until your hips are below your knee. Keep your weight on your heels as you drive up.

48 Straight-arm crunch

TARGET Upper abs

DIFFICULTY RATING ⊕⊕⊕⊕⊙

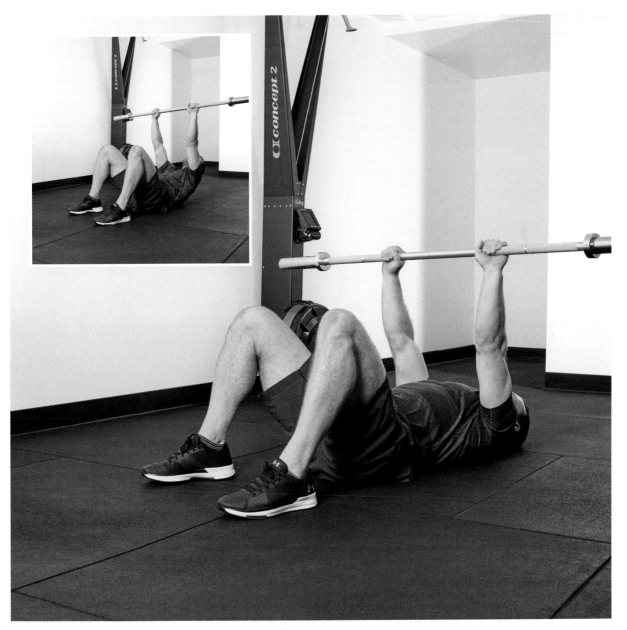

WHY This is a challenging move that will help you to build strong abs. It will also help to strengthen and stabilise the small muscles of the shoulder joint, which will have a beneficial effect on your bench pressing ability.

HOW Lie on the floor with your knees bent and hold the barbell, with your arms straight, above your chest. Keeping your arms vertical, contract your abs to raise your head and shoulders off the floor.

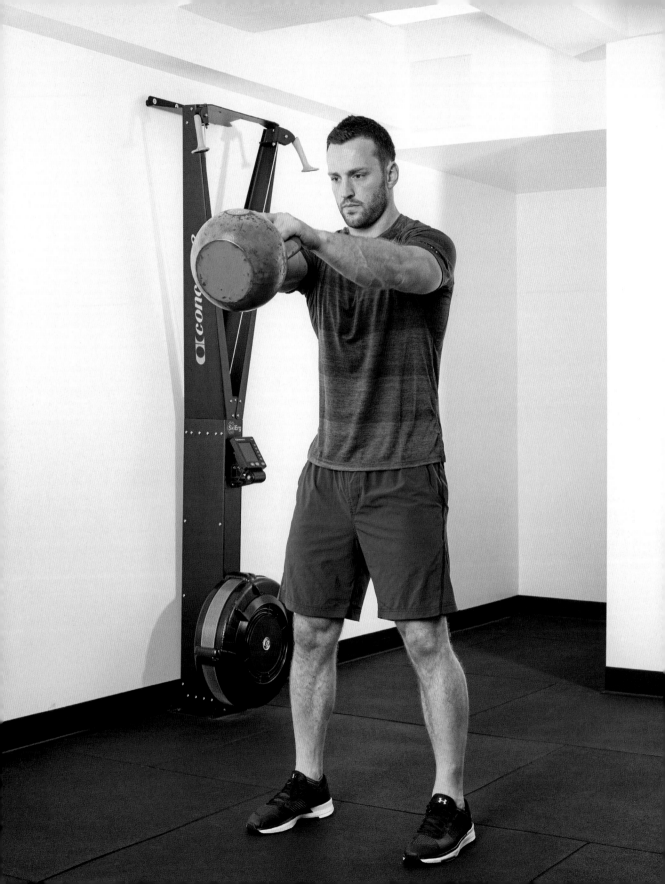

KETTLEBELL EXERCISES

49 Angel press

TARGET Upper abs

DIFFICULTY RATING ●●●●○

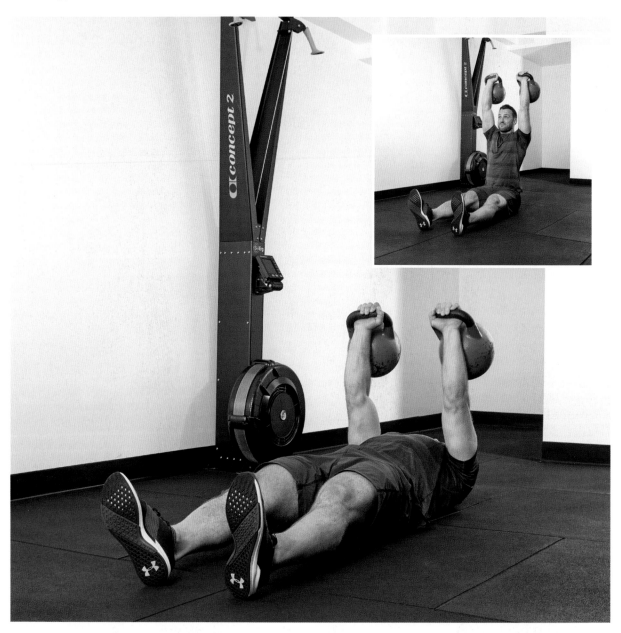

WHY This is an advanced abs move so you may want to save it until you have built some solid foundations. The trick to making it effective is to control the lowering phase, rather than just flopping back onto the floor.

HOW Lie on your back holding two kettlebells with straight arms above your shoulders. Contract your abs to crunch up and raise your head and shoulders off the floor, then lower slowly back to the start.

50 Bent press

TARGET Shoulders, triceps, side abs and core

DIFFICULTY RATING ●●●●○

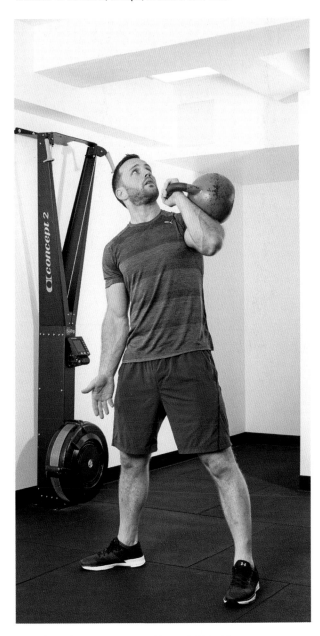

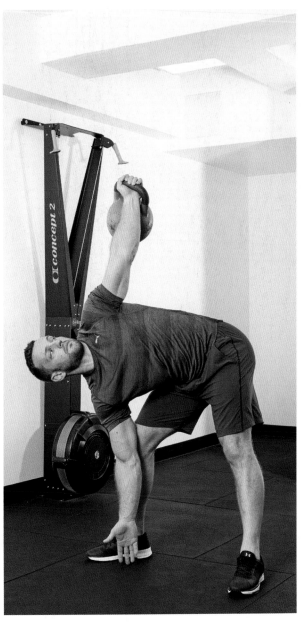

WHY The idea is not to press the weight but to support it as you get underneath it, which provides a real test of core and shoulder stability.

HOW Hold the bell at shoulder height, then bend away from it while your upper arm is in contact with your body. Then start pressing, and keep lowering your torso until your arm is straight. Then straighten up to return to the start.

51 Figure of eight

TARGET Side abs

DIFFICULTY RATING ●●●○○

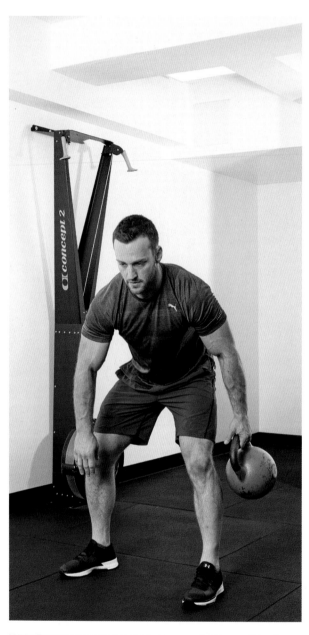

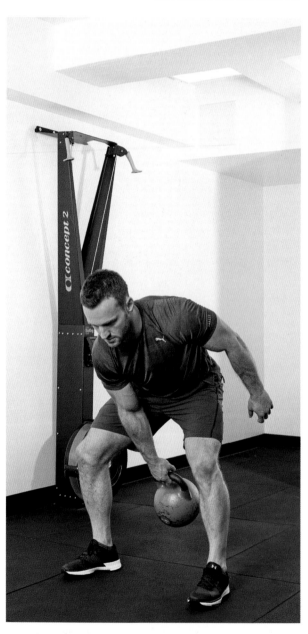

WHY This is as much a test of your coordination as it is of your core control. The weight is constantly moving so you can't switch off, either physically or mentally, for a second.

HOW Swing the weight out in front of you, then pass it back between your legs and switch hands. With the other hand, swing the weight back, out and around your other leg, then pass it through your legs again to continue the pattern.

52 Halo

TARGET Abs and core

DIFFICULTY RATING ⊙⊙⊙⊙⊙

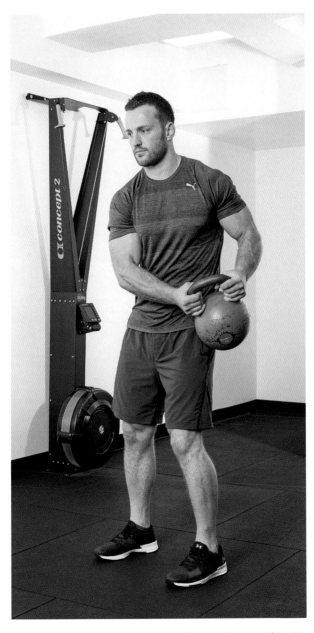

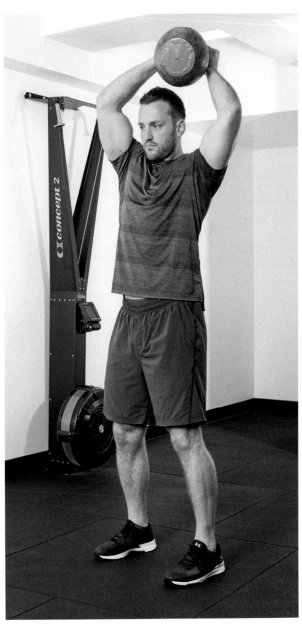

WHY This move engages your shoulders and core, making it the ideal warm-up when done light – or a fat-burning finisher when used alongside other kettlebell exercises.

HOW Holding the kettlebell by the handle with both hands, manoeuvre it around your head, bending your elbows as it passes behind you for the maximum range of motion. You'll feel this one in your obliques if you do it right.

53 Plank pass

TARGET Abs and core

DIFFICULTY RATING ●●○○○

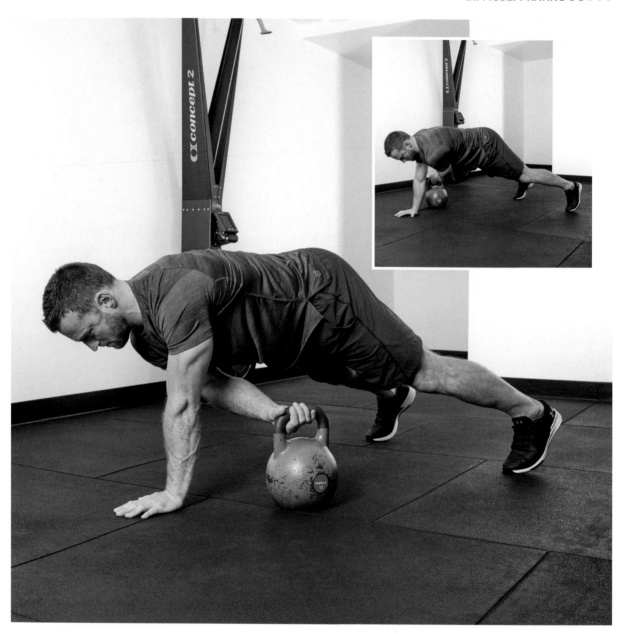

WHY Once you can do the plank for at least two minutes, this variation adds instability and a twisting motion, hitting your core from every angle. You can also do it with a dumbbell or sandbag.

HOW Get into a straight-arm plank position with the kettlebell underneath you. Grasp it with one hand and pull it across your body, then change hands and repeat on the other side. Try to keep your torso straight throughout.

54 Renegade row

TARGET Abs and core

DIFFICULTY RATING ●●●○○

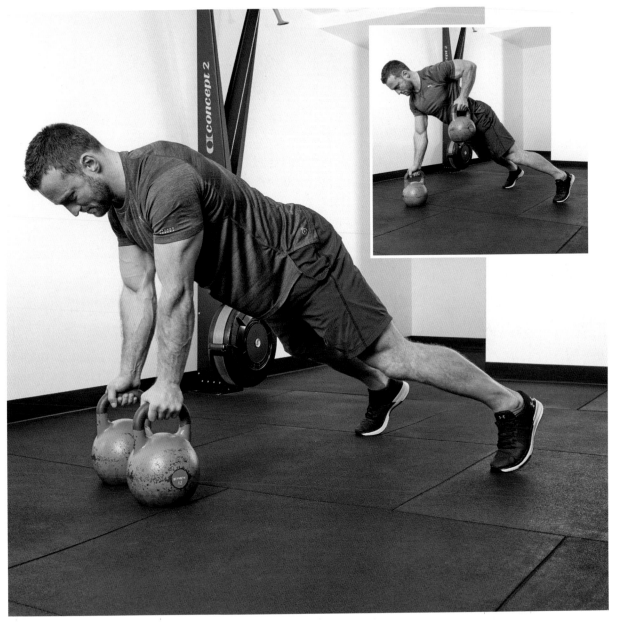

WHY This move combines stability with pulling, so it'll build your core as well as your back. It's tempting to twist to one side as the reps get tougher, but the more you can stay parallel, the harder you'll work your abs.

HOW Start in a press-up position holding a pair of kettlebells. Do a press-up. At the top of the move, row one bell up (so that your thumb touches your armpit) and down, then the other.

55 Rolling thunder

TARGET Chest, abs and core

DIFFICULTY RATING ●●●○○

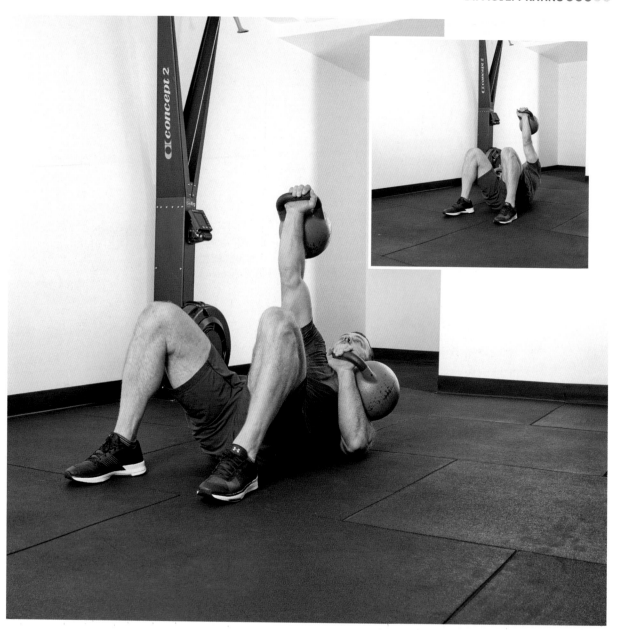

WHY This move uses full-body coordination while forcing your core to work under load, building real-world strength that'll be useful in almost any sport. It'll also give your shoulders some much-needed stability work.

HOW Lie with a kettlebell in each hand, keeping your knees bent. Press one kettlebell up, rolling to that side and bringing your shoulder off the ground. As you lower the first kettlebell, roll the other way and press the other one.

56 Round the world

TARGET Abs, lower back and core

DIFFICULTY RATING ●●○○○

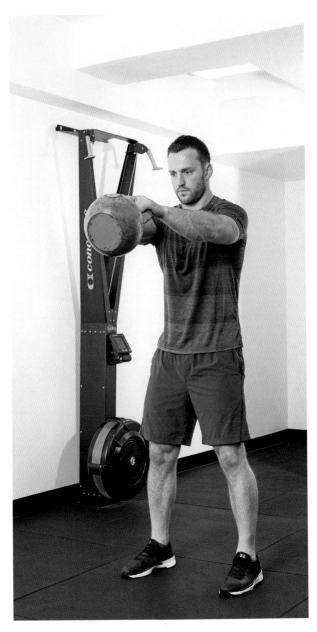
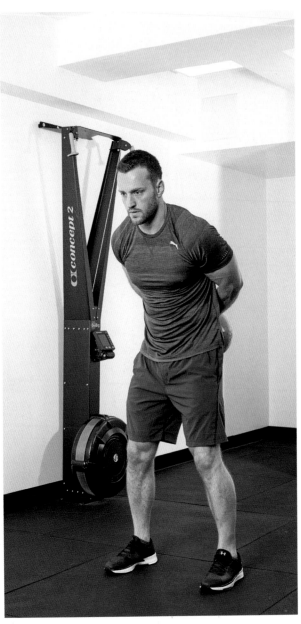

WHY Done at speed, this move gets all your core muscles firing, making it a good warm-up (done light) or a good finisher (done heavy, in conjunction with other moves). It'll also work your grip, if you keep at it for a while.

HOW Stand tall with the kettlebell in one hand, then swing it around your body, switching hands as it passes in front of and behind you.

57 Side press

TARGET Shoulders, triceps and side abs

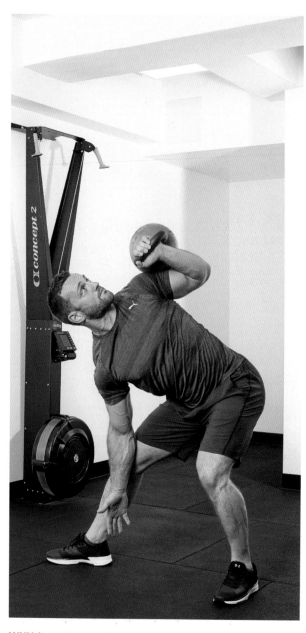

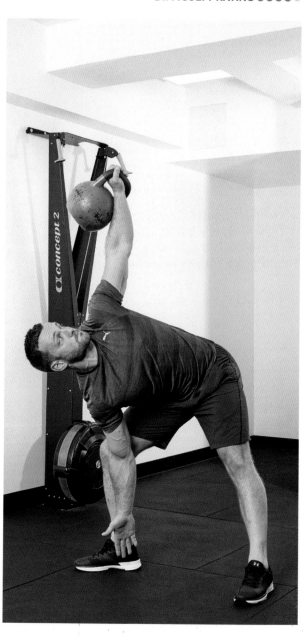

WHY As well as working your core, this lift allows you to handle significantly more weight than a traditional overhead press, as your press should be stronger out to the side than straight overhead.

HOW Take a fairly wide stance and lead to the side, with that foot pointed in the direction you're leaning. Press the kettlebell upwards until your arm is straight, then lower under control.

58 Snatch

TARGET Whole body

DIFFICULTY RATING ●●●●○

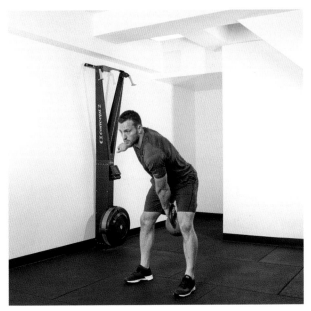

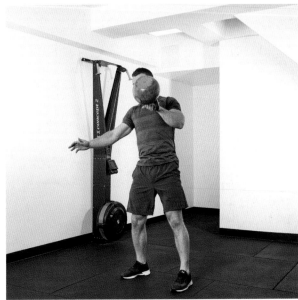

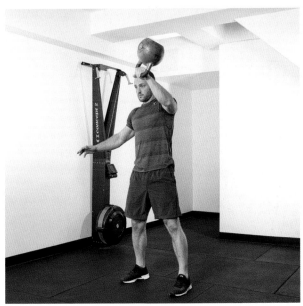

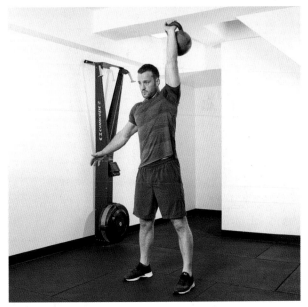

WHY Though it's tricky to master, the snatch is worth it – this full-body test of coordination demands serious lung power when done properly.

HOW Swing the kettlebell between your legs with one hand, then pop your hips forwards to drive it up. When it gets to chest level, punch your hand forwards and catch it on your forearm, bringing it overhead.

59 Turkish get-up

TARGET Whole body

DIFFICULTY RATING ●●●●○

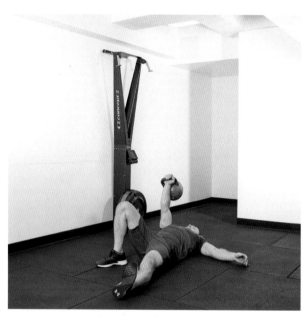

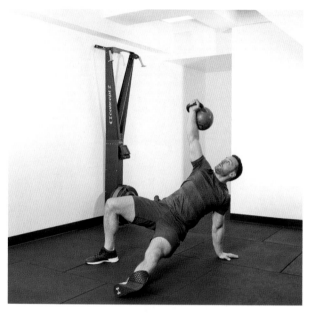

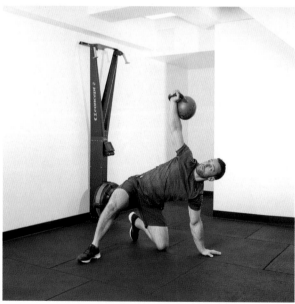

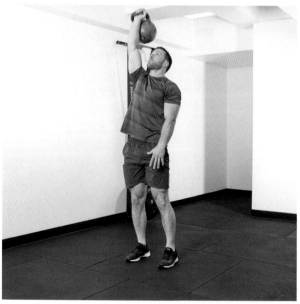

WHY This move builds strength and balance through your whole body, as well as teaching you to create tension and stability in a variety of positions.

HOW Lie on your back with the kettlebell held up. Supporting yourself on the other arm, plant the foot on the kettlebell side on the floor. Sweep your other leg back and plant the knee on the floor. Stand up with the kettlebell overhead.

60 Windmill

TARGET Side abs

DIFFICULTY RATING ⦿⦿⦿⦿⦾

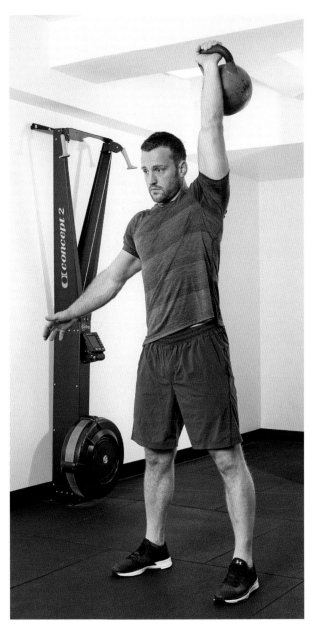
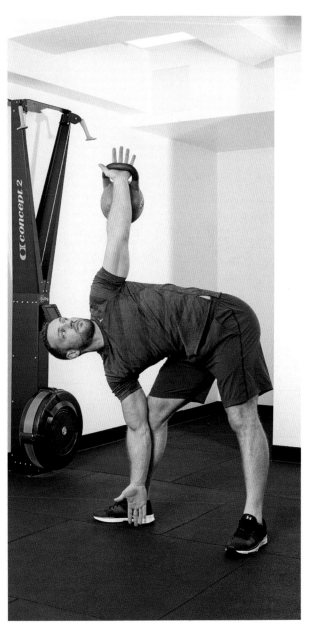

WHY This move targets your obliques and works on your coordination. It's also a great dynamic hamstring stretch – ideal for warming up on a big deadlift day.

HOW Stand holding a kettlebell overhead, then lean to one side so that your free hand travels down your leg. Keep your arm and back straight throughout.

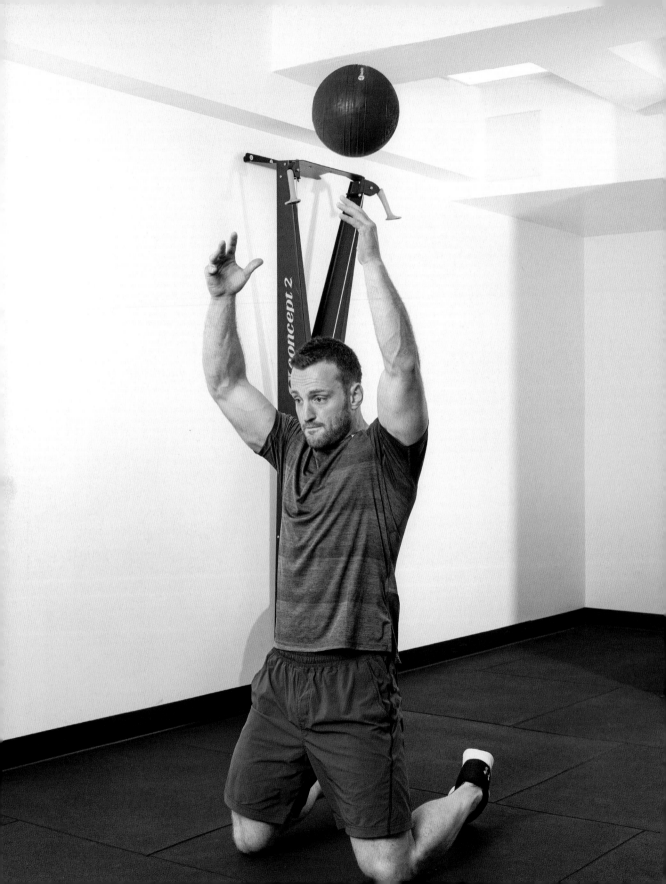

MEDICINE BALL EXERCISES

61 Crunch

TARGET Upper abs

DIFFICULTY RATING ●●○○○

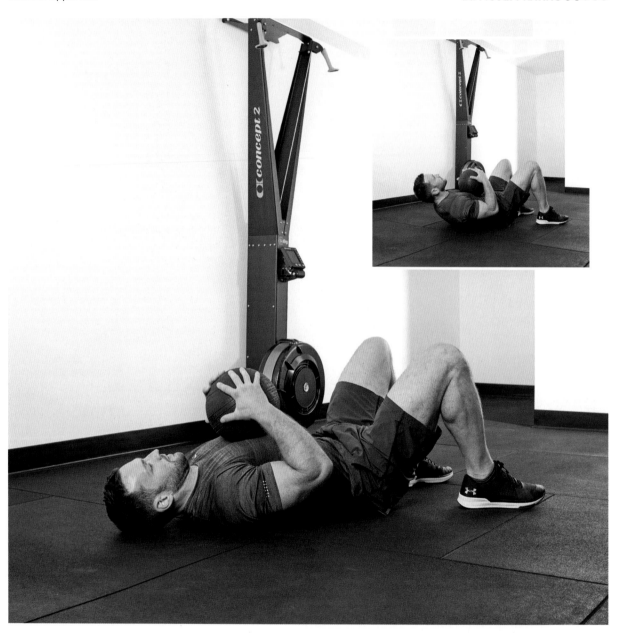

WHY Adding resistance to the classic crunch exercise makes it harder, so this is a good option once you're past the beginner stage or if you're doing a medicine ball circuit.

HOW Lie on your back with knees bent, holding a med ball against your chest. Contract your upper abs to raise your torso off the ground, pause at the top, then lower back to the start.

62 Feet on ball press-up

TARGET Abs and core

DIFFICULTY RATING ●●●●○

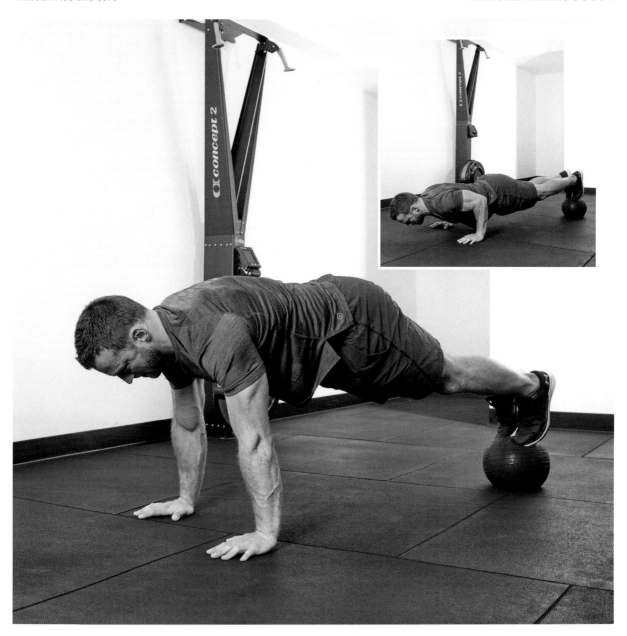

WHY This is a really tough version of the press-up so don't worry if you can't do many reps or even do it at all. You might want to start by taking a little time to get comfortable in the start position.

HOW Start with your feet on a med ball and your hands on the floor directly below your shoulders, body in a straight line from head to heels. Bend your elbows to lower to the floor, then press back up.

63 Lying knee raise

TARGET Lower abs

WHY The lying knee raise works your lower abs and the added resistance will make the move harder, so use it once you can easily do sets of 20 reps without a weight.

HOW Lie flat on your back with arms by your sides holding a med ball between your knees. Contract your lower abs to raise your knees towards your chest. Pause at the top, then return to the start.

64 Lying leg raise

TARGET Lower abs   **DIFFICULTY RATING** ⊕⊕⊕⊕⊕

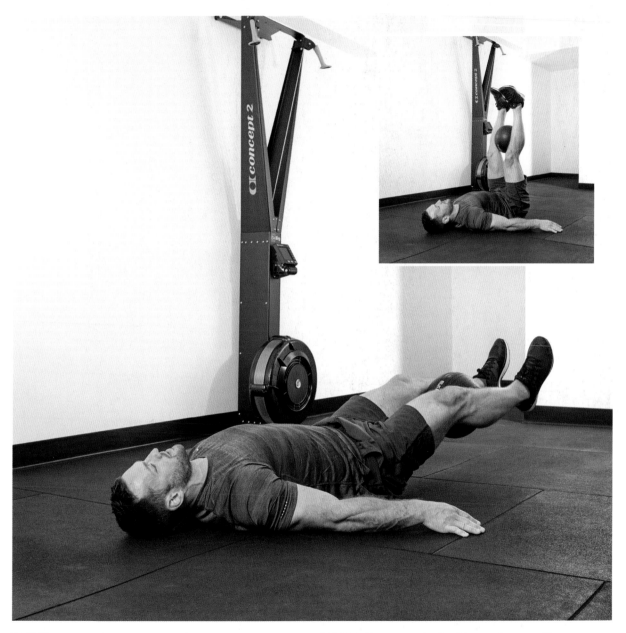

WHY This is a tough move because the weight is so far away from your body. Start light and increase the load as you progress. Make sure you don't excessively arch your back at any point during the rep.

HOW Lie flat on your back with arms by your sides holding a med ball held between your calves or feet. Contract your lower abs to raise your legs as high as you can. Pause at the top, then return to the start.

65 Overhead throw

TARGET Abs and core

DIFFICULTY RATING ●●○○○

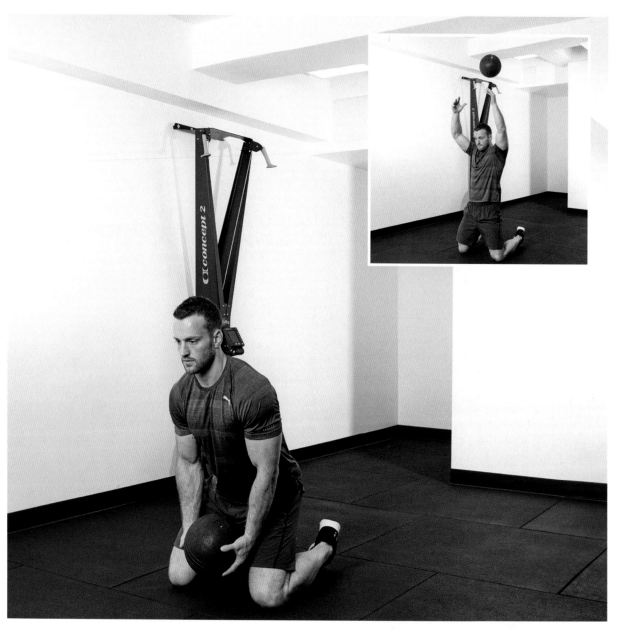

WHY Medicine ball throws are a great way of training because they allow you to work at maximum intensity but are relatively safe to perform.

HOW Hold a med ball in both hands in front of you, then throw it up and over your head. Just make sure there's no-one behind you.

66 Passing press-up

TARGET Chest, triceps, abs and core

DIFFICULTY RATING ●●●○○

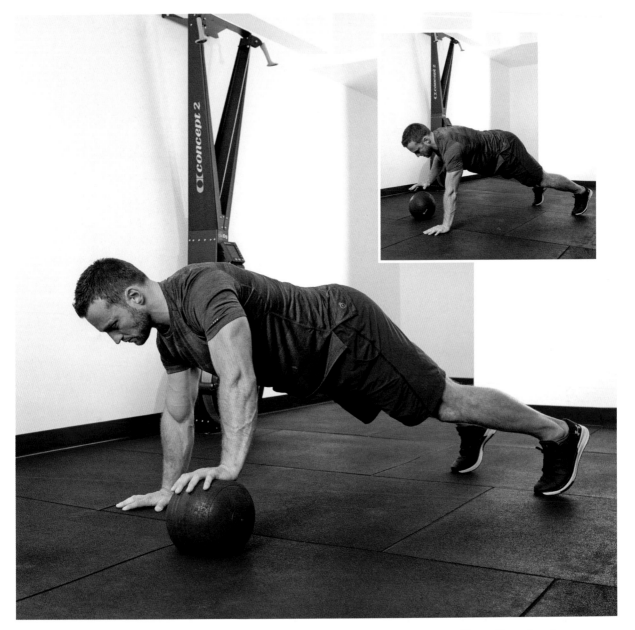

WHY This dynamic exercise will keep your core engaged and your balance tested throughout the set. It also develops your chest muscles.

HOW Start in a press-up position with one hand on a med ball. Perform a press-up, then roll the ball towards your other hand. Re-set your hands and perform a press-up with the other hand on the ball.

67 Plank

TARGET Abs and core

DIFFICULTY RATING ●●●○○

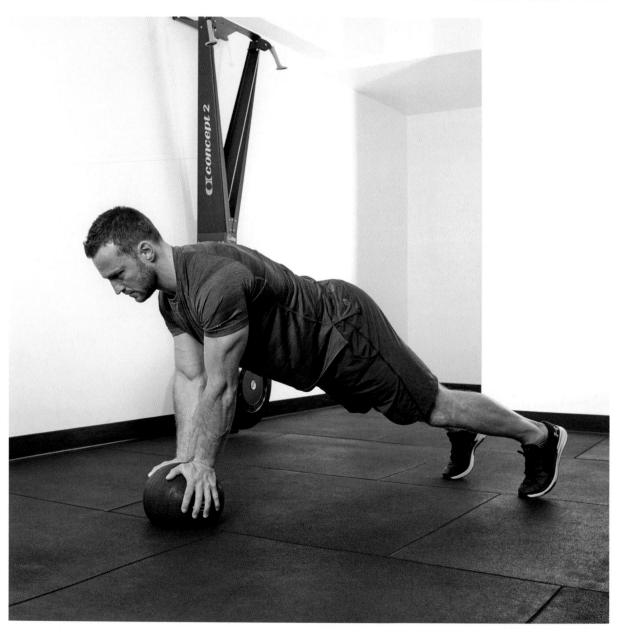

WHY Once you have mastered the standard plank (see p22) you can begin to experiment with more difficult variations of the exercise. This move is also a good warm-up for the medicine ball press-up (opposite).

HOW With arms straight, place your hands either side of a med ball and hold your body in a straight line from head to heels, head looking straight down. Brace your abs to hold this position without letting your hips sag.

68 Press-up

TARGET Chest, triceps, abs and core

DIFFICULTY RATING ⊕⊕⊕⊕⊕

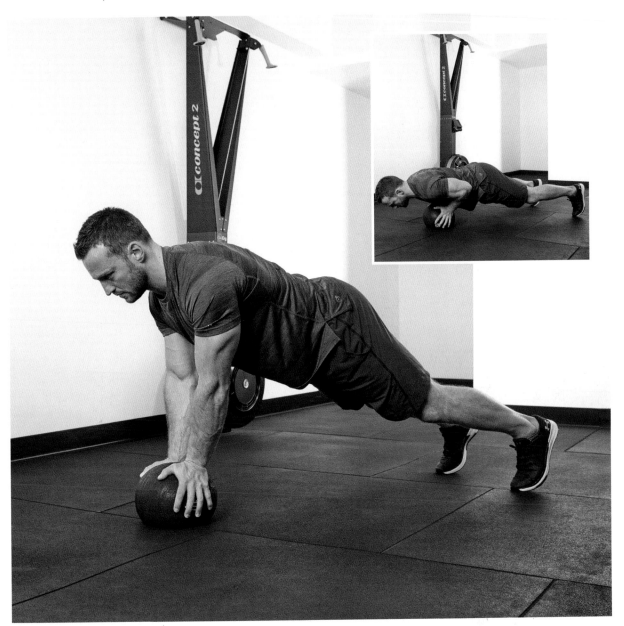

WHY This is one of the most difficult press-up variations you can do. The fact that you're on an unstable surface makes it hard but the close position of your hands means that it is your triceps, rather than your chest, that power the move.

HOW Start with both hands on the ball and your body in a straight line from head to heels. Bend at the elbows to lower your chest towards the floor, then press back up. Ensure that your elbows don't flare out during the rep.

69 Russian twist

TARGET Side abs

DIFFICULTY RATING ●●○○○

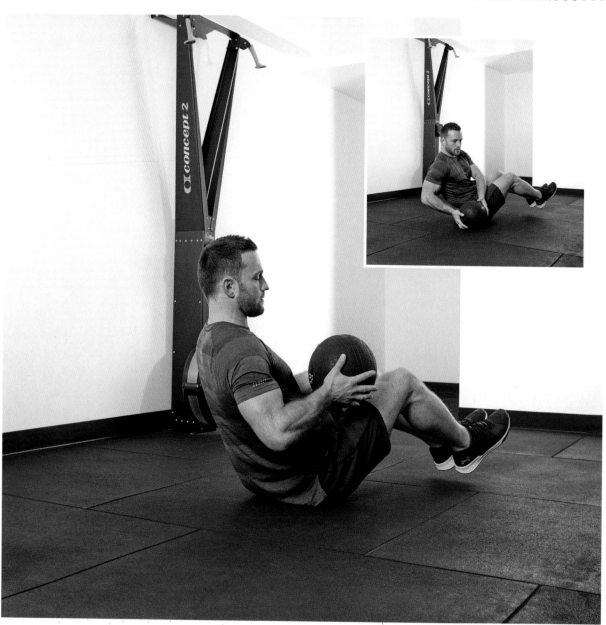

WHY You can do Russian twists with dumbbells or weight plates but the medicine ball is a good option because they are easy to hold, so you can concentrate on the quality of abdominal contraction.

HOW Sit with your torso at a 45° angle to the floor and knees bent, holding a medicine ball in both hands in front of you. Twist to one side, then come back to the centre and twist to the other side.

70 Slam

TARGET Abs and core

DIFFICULTY RATING ●●○○○

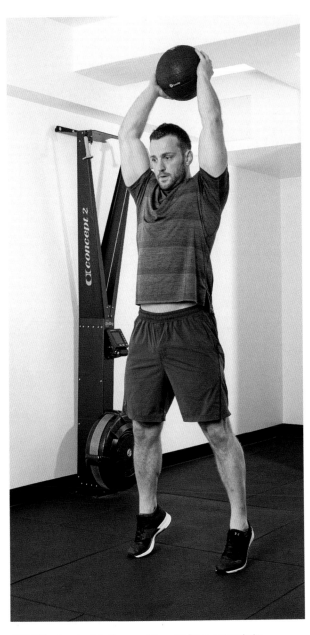 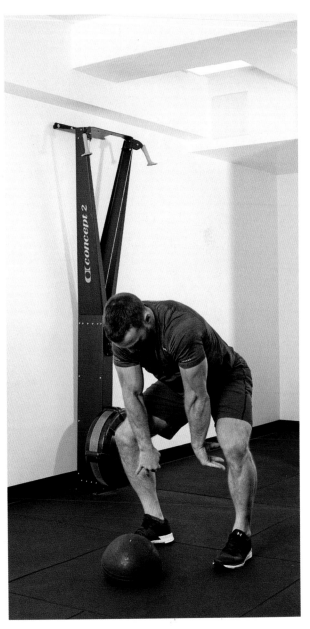

WHY The key to this thoroughly satisfying move is to perform it as explosively as possible. Just letting the ball fall to the floor won't have the same benefit.

HOW Stand holding a medicine ball to your chest, then raise it overhead, rise onto your toes and slam it down powerfully to the floor. Catch it and repeat the exercise.

71 Sledgehammer

TARGET Abs and core

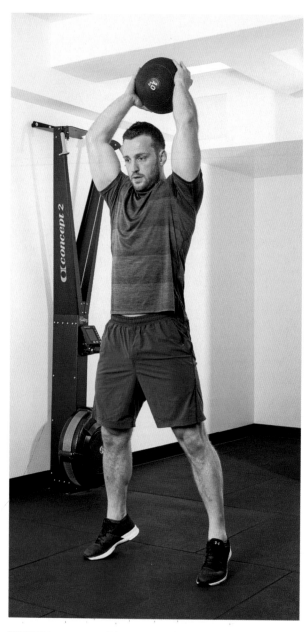

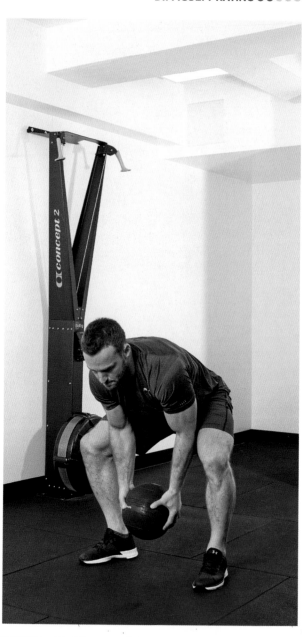

WHY This move combines some of the benefits of the overhead throw and the slam. You hold on to the ball as you raise it and lower it so you also have to control the deceleration phase of the movement.

HOW Stand holding a medicine ball to your chest. Explosively raise it overhead, then bring it down in front of you while simultaneously lowering into a squat. Rise and repeat the exercise.

72 Side throw

TARGET Side abs

DIFFICULTY RATING ●●●○○

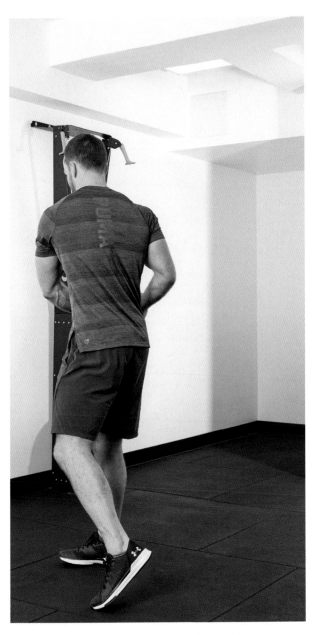

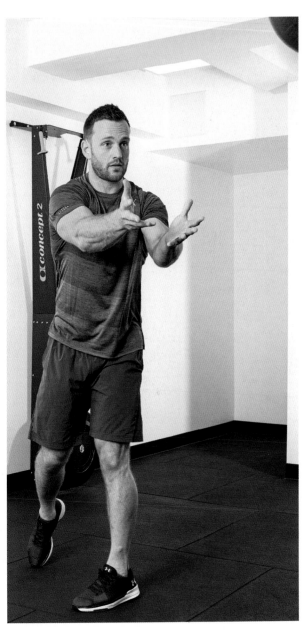

WHY Not all throws have to be up and down. This side throw is an excellent way of training your side abs and will be especially useful if you play rugby.

HOW Stand up straight holding a medicine ball. Swing it to one side slightly, then throw it as explosively as possible to the other side. Reset and repeat the exercise on the other side.

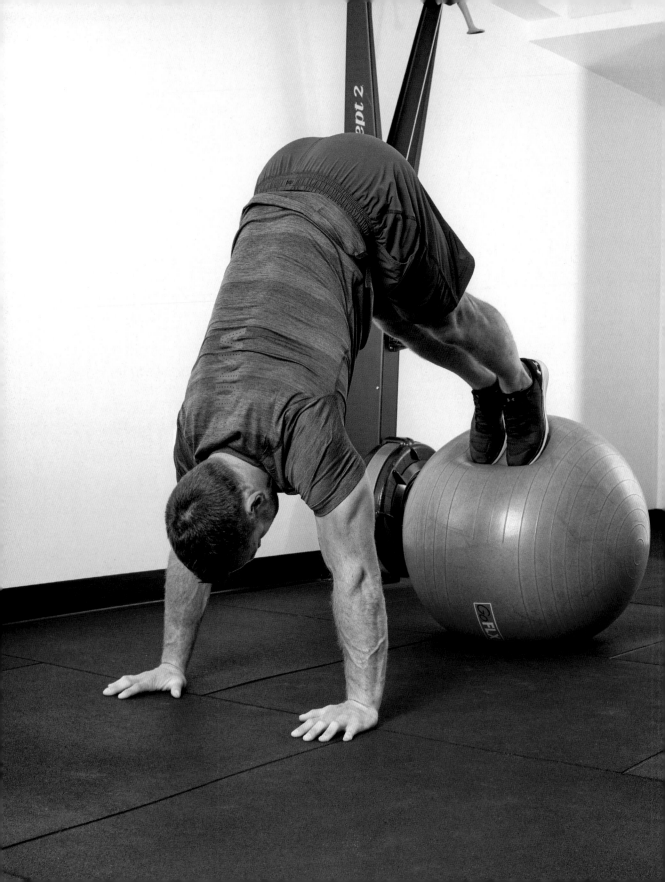

GYM BALL EXERCISES

73 Crunch

TARGET Upper abs

DIFFICULTY RATING ❍❍❍❍❍

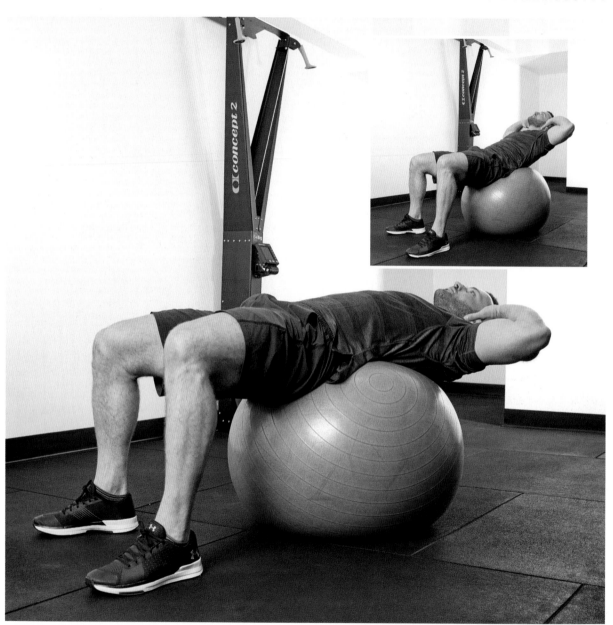

WHY Performing a crunch on a gym ball is arguably the most effective way of doing the exercise because you can start with your abs in extension, which improves the muscle contraction as you crunch.

HOW Lie on your back on a gym ball with feet flat on the floor and fingers touching your temples. Contract your upper abs to raise your torso off the ball, pause at the top, then lower back to the start.

74 Crunch twist

TARGET Upper and side abs

DIFFICULTY RATING ●●●○○

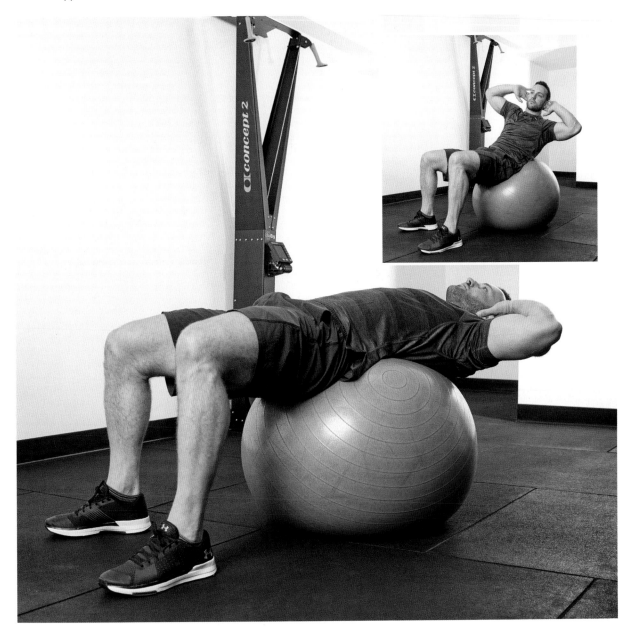

WHY This move may look simple but it is deceptively difficult and, as such, is also very effective because it takes a lot of core control and balance to avoid falling off the ball.

HOW Lie on your back on a gym ball with feet flat on the floor and fingers at your temples. Contract your upper abs to raise your torso off the ball, then rotate to one side. Pause at the top, lower back to the start, then repeat to the other side.

75 Decline plank

TARGET Abs and core

DIFFICULTY RATING ●●●○○

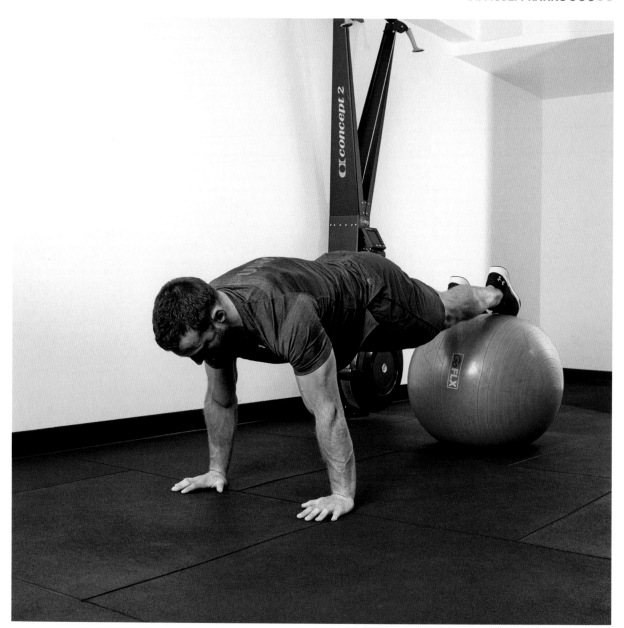

WHY Once you master the standard plank you'll need to make it more challenging to get the benefit of the exercise, and this variation provides extra instability.

HOW Hold your body in a straight line from head to heels with your elbows directly beneath your shoulders and both feet on a gym ball. Brace your abs to hold this position and don't let your hips sag.

76 Incline plank

TARGET Abs and core

DIFFICULTY RATING ⦿⦿⦿⦿○

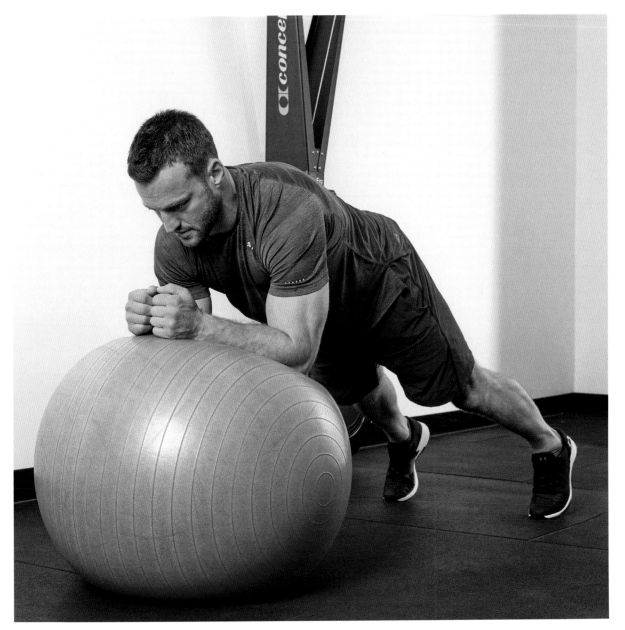

WHY Once you've mastered the decline plank (see opposite) you can move on to this variation. Placing your arms on the ball is a lot harder than doing it with your feet or legs on the ball.

HOW Hold your body in a straight line from head to heels with your elbows on a gym ball directly beneath your shoulders. Brace your abs to hold this position and don't let your hips sag.

77 Jackknife

TARGET Abs and core

DIFFICULTY RATING ●●●○○

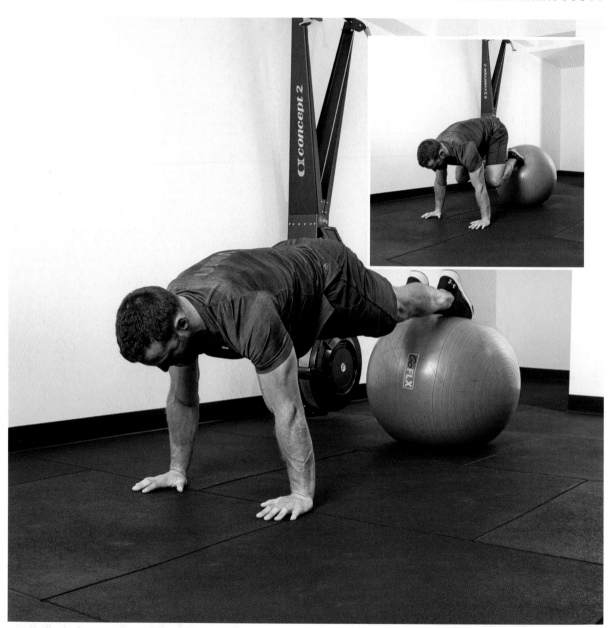

WHY Any move that brings your knees up to your chest will work your hard-to-target lower abs. This move does that while providing a test of your overall core strength.

HOW Hold your body in a straight line from head to heels with your elbows directly beneath your shoulders and both feet on a gym ball, then draw your knees in towards your chest. Pause, then return to the start position.

78 Jackknife twist

TARGET Abs and core

DIFFICULTY RATING ●●●●○

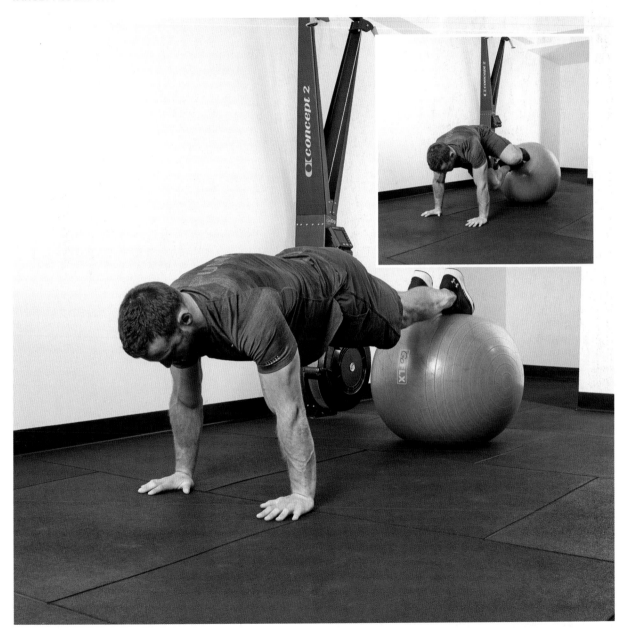

WHY This exercise offer similar benefits to the standard jackknife but the twist element means you will also challenge your side abs.

HOW Hold your body in a straight line from head to heels with both feet on a gym ball, then draw your knees in towards your chest and use your abs to rotate to one side. Pause, then rotate to the other side.

79 Passing V-up

TARGET Abs and core

DIFFICULTY RATING ●●●●○

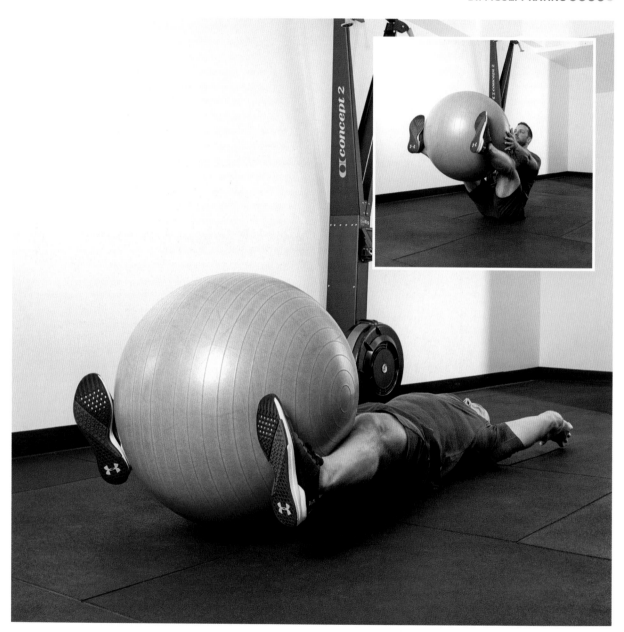

WHY There's no way to do this move in a half-hearted manner so you need to focus on a good-quality contraction of your abs. It's also a real skill to time the exercise correctly so that you meet in the middle.

HOW Lie on your back with a gym ball between your legs. Contract your abs to bring your feet and hands up to meet each other in the middle and pass the ball from feet to hands. Continue passing it back and forth.

80 Pike

TARGET Abs and core

DIFFICULTY RATING ●●●○○

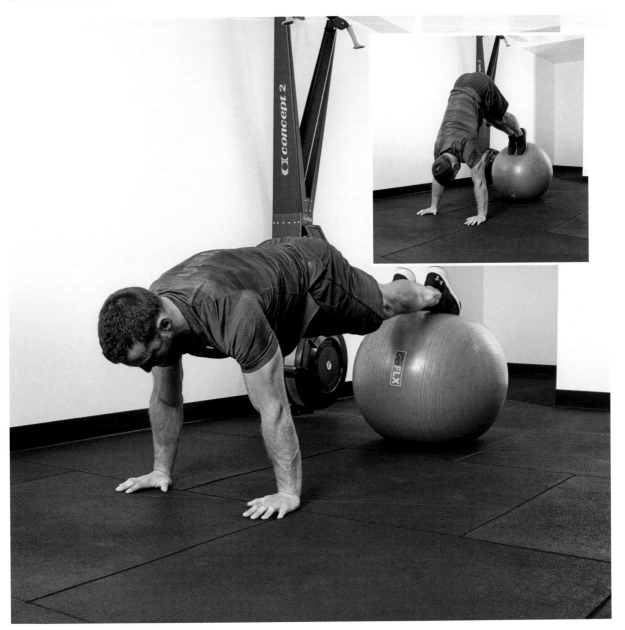

WHY This gymnastics-style exercise is fun to do and also more accessible than it looks. The hip hinge and crunch is an effective way of improving the way your abs and pelvis move together.

HOW Hold your body in a straight line from head to heels and both feet on a gym ball. Contract your abs to draw your feet in towards your hands so your body forms a V-shape. Pause at the top, then lower back to the start.

81 Press-up

TARGET Chest, abs and core

DIFFICULTY RATING ⦿⦿⦿⦿⦾

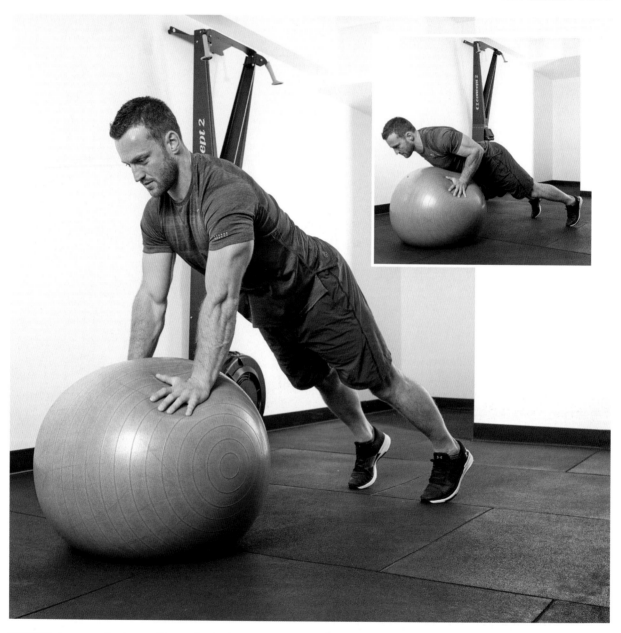

WHY This is an excellent way of improving both your core stability and also your shoulder stability. It's a tough move so make sure your reps are slow and controlled.

HOW Start with your hands on a gym ball below your chest with your arms straight and your body straight from head to heels. Bend your elbows to lower your chest towards the ball, then push back up.

82 Roll-out

TARGET Abs and core

DIFFICULTY RATING ●●○○○

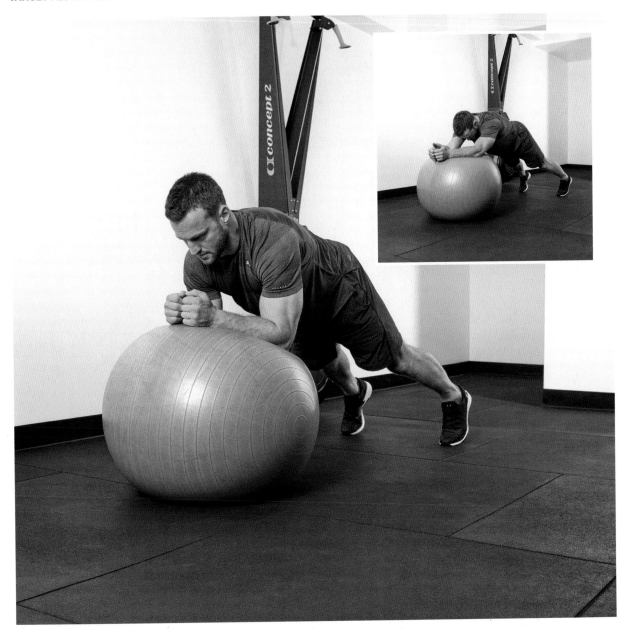

WHY The movement involved in a roll-out is very effective for building abs strength and improving posture, but the barbell version (see p61) is difficult for beginners to master – this is an accessible alternative.

HOW Place both elbows on a gym ball and keep your body straight. Brace your core and roll the ball away from your knees as far you can. Pause, then reverse the movement back to the start.

83 Russian twist

TARGET Side abs

DIFFICULTY RATING ●●●○○

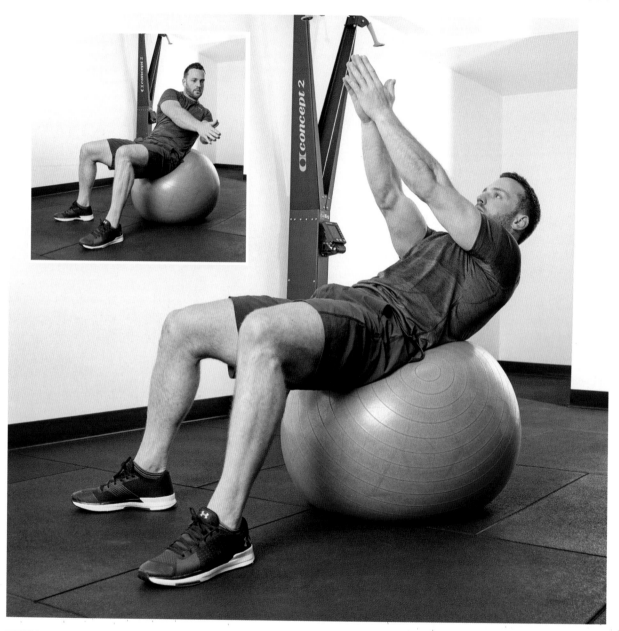

WHY As with the gym ball crunch twist, using a ball to do a variation on an easy move makes it more of a challenge. Lower to the side as far as you can while remaining in control of the movement.

HOW Lie with your back supported on a gym ball with arms straight above your chest and hands together. Rotate your torso to one side to lower your hands. Pause, then return to the start and lower them to the other side.

84 Toe touch decline plank

TARGET Abs and core

DIFFICULTY RATING ●●●●○

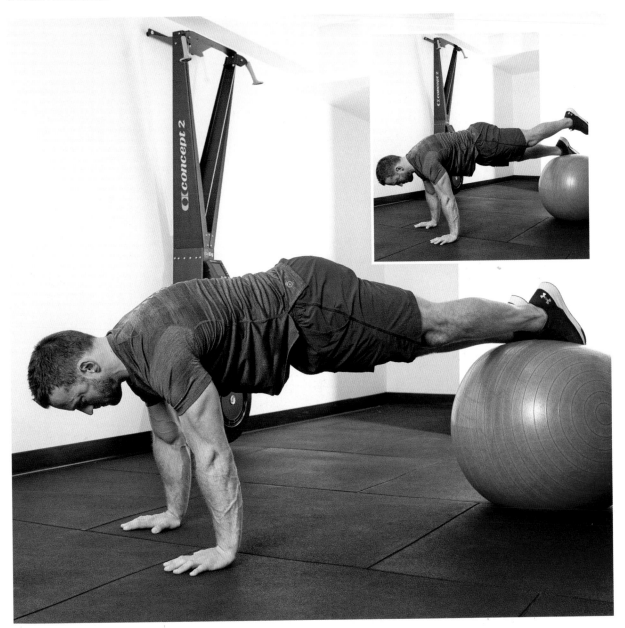

WHY This is a really tricky move but it's worth doing because it gives you the ability to switch on your core while also moving your limbs in a specific way, which translates well to sporting challenges.

HOW Hold your body in a straight line with both feet on a gym ball. Brace your abs to hold this position without letting your hips sag, then lift one foot and touch it to the floor. Return to the start, then repeat with the other foot.

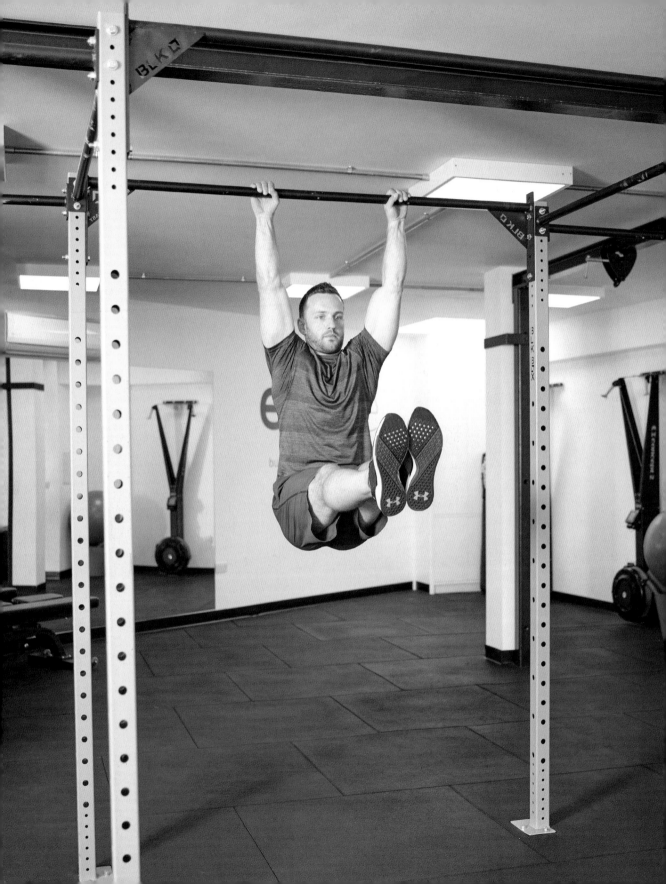

PULL-UP BAR EXERCISES

85 Garhammer raise

TARGET Lower abs

DIFFICULTY RATING ●●●○○

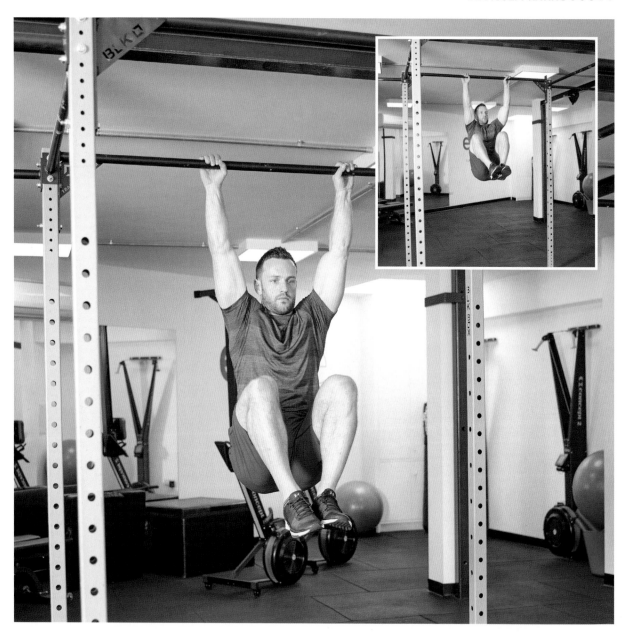

WHY This variation of the knee raise (see p110) keeps tension on your lower abs throughout, not letting them relax like 'easier' variations. Keep the form strict and you'll grow.

HOW Hang from a pull-up bar and raise your knees to hip height. Then raise your knees as high as possible, then lower them to hip height again. Keep constant tension in your abs throughout.

86 Knee hold

TARGET Lower abs

DIFFICULTY RATING ●●○○○

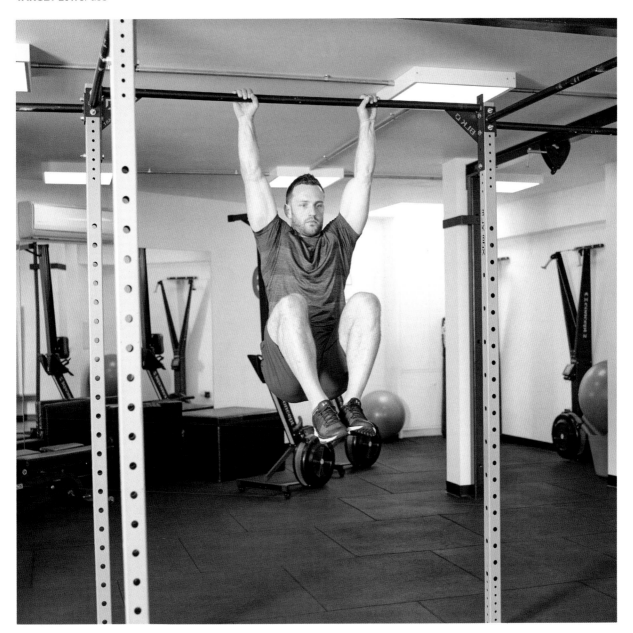

WHY It's generally quite difficult to contract your lower abs, but this exercise is an accessible and effective way of targeting that portion of your midsection.

HOW Hang from a bar with your body straight, using an overhand grip. Keeping your knees bent, use your lower abs to raise your knees to hip height. Hold that position.

87 Knee raise

TARGET Lower abs

DIFFICULTY RATING ⦿○○○○

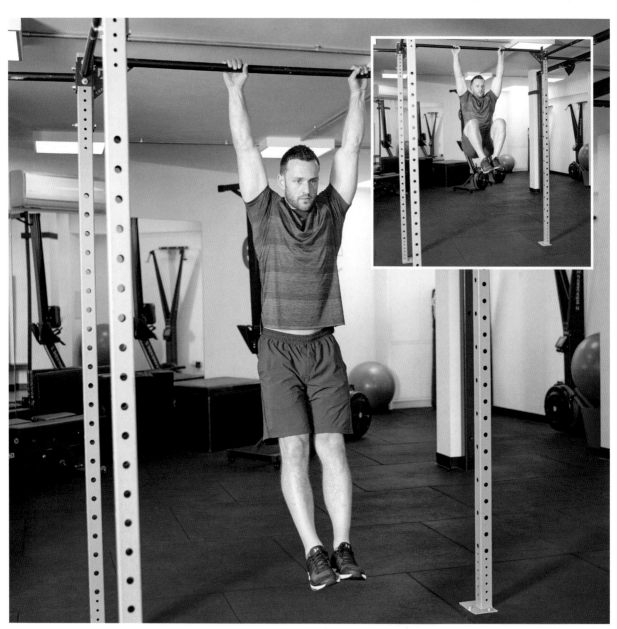

WHY One of the most basic but best abs moves you can do, the knee raise also challenges your grip and forearms. Do it slowly for great results. If your grip's limiting the number of reps you can do, try using straps for your final couple of sets.

HOW Hang from a bar with your body straight, using an overhand grip. Keeping your knees bent, use your lower abs to raise your knees to hip height. Lower under control.

88 Knee raise twist

TARGET Lower and side abs

DIFFICULTY RATING ●●○○○

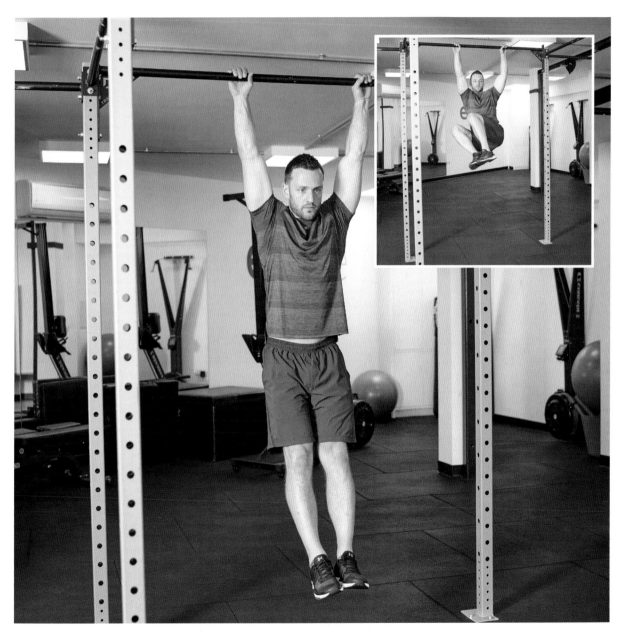

WHY Adding a twist to the knee raise gets your obliques involved in the move, as well as forcing you to focus on form. Again, keep the move slow and controlled for the greatest possible benefit.

HOW Hang from a bar with your body straight, using an overhand grip. Keeping your knees bent, raise them to hip height. As your knees approach the top of the move, twist to the side – you should feel this in your obliques.

89 Leg hold

TARGET Abs and core

DIFFICULTY RATING ●●●○○

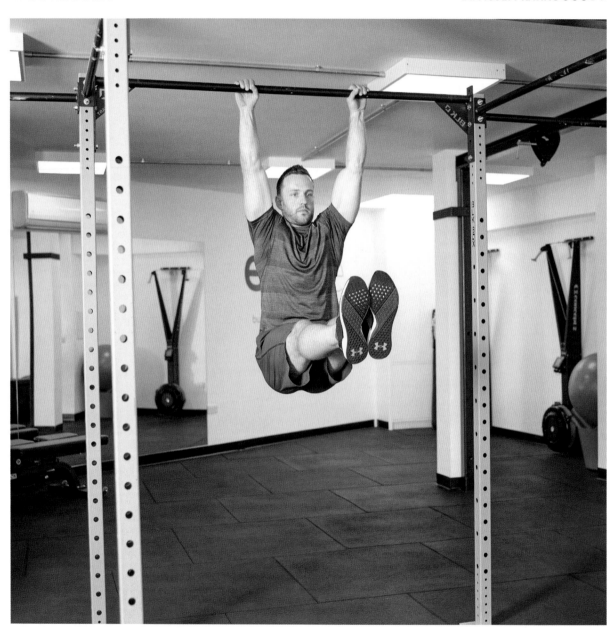

WHY Think of this as an upgraded version of the knee hold (see p109). It too mainly works your lower abs but it is so challenging that your entire core and abs will need to be activated to hold your body in position.

HOW Hang from a bar with your body straight. Keeping your legs straight, use your lower abs to raise them until they're parallel with the floor. Hold that position.

90 Leg raise

TARGET Abs and core

DIFFICULTY RATING ●●●○○

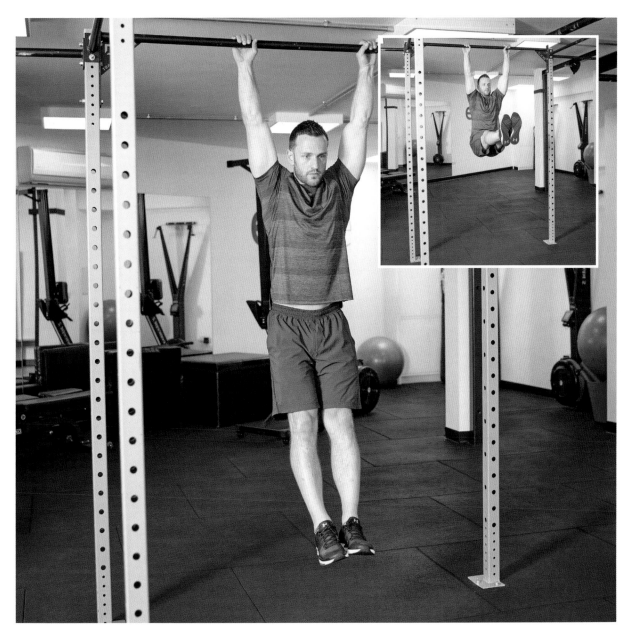

WHY Once you can do ten knee raises with good form, it's time to graduate. The greater leverages involved make this a much tougher move.

HOW Hang from a bar with your body straight. Keeping your legs straight, use your lower abs to raise them until they're parallel with the floor. Pause, then lower under control.

91 L-sit pull-up

TARGET Back, biceps, abs and core

DIFFICULTY RATING ●●●●○

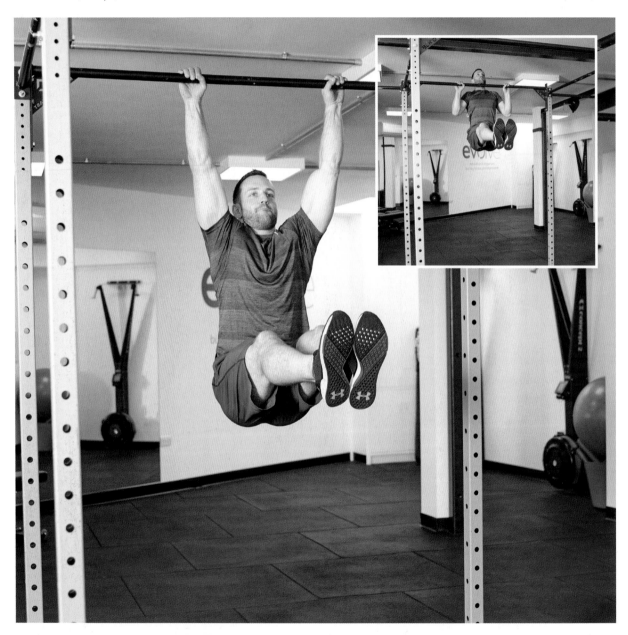

WHY As well as working your abs, the L-sit pull-up puts more emphasis on your lats. If you find 'unlocking' your shoulders at the bottom difficult, build up with L-sit hangs.

HOW Hang from a bar with an overhand grip and bring your legs up until they're parallel to the floor. Brace your core to remain in an L-shape as you pull up until your chin's over the bar.

92 Windscreen wiper

TARGET Abs and core

DIFFICULTY RATING ❍❍❍❍❍

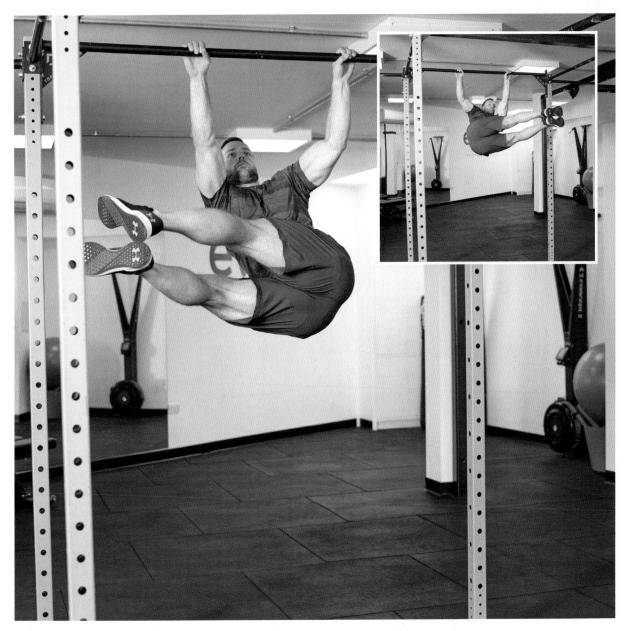

WHY There are a couple of reasons you might want to do this exercise. The first is if you want to give your side abs a real challenge. The second is if you want to show off – it looks really impressive.

HOW Hang from a bar using an overhand grip, then bring your feet up to the bar with your legs straight. Lower your feet to one side, then bring them back to the middle and lower to the other side.

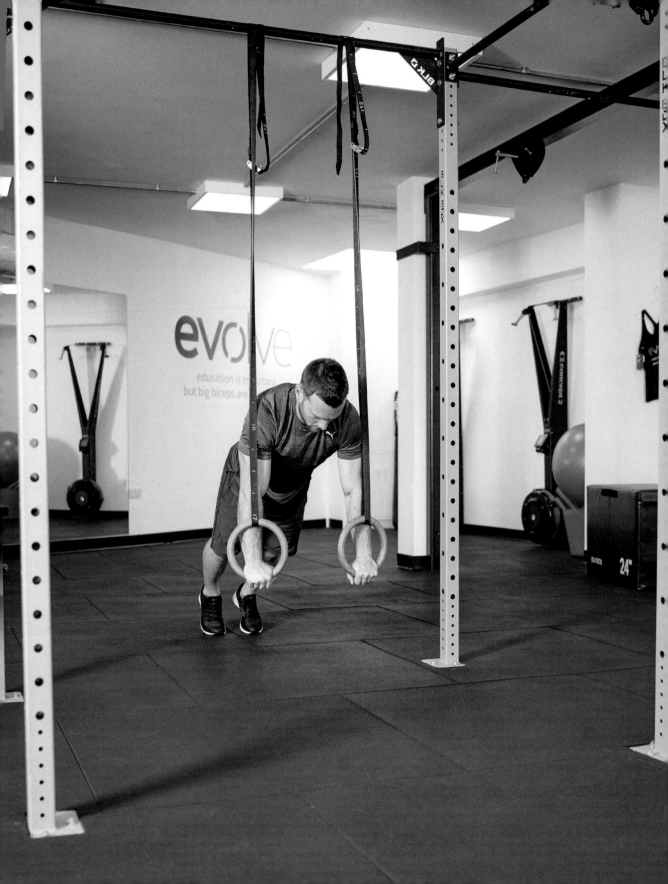

SUSPENSION EXERCISES

93 Flye

TARGET Chest, abs and core

DIFFICULTY RATING ●●○○○

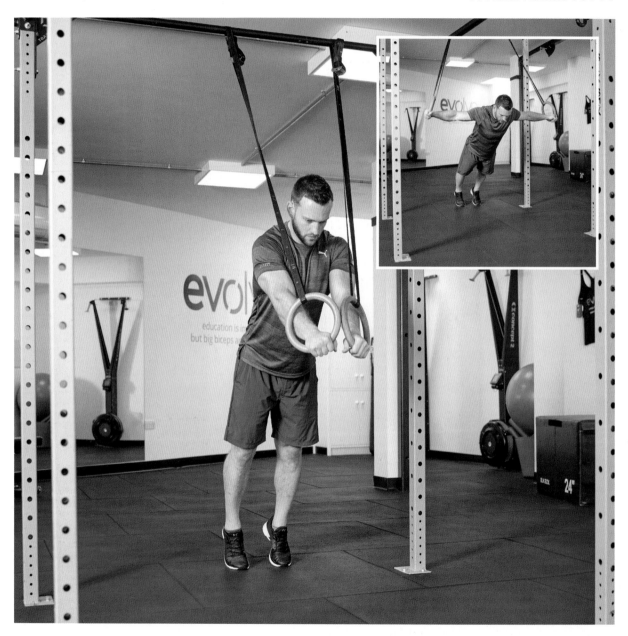

WHY This move does put your pecs under constant tension while also providing a jolt to your core and biceps. Superset it with ring press-ups (see p124) for a guaranteed chest-builder.

HOW Stand tall holding the rings with your palms facing in. Lean forwards, allowing your arms to come out to your sides to form a T-shape, keeping a slight bend in your elbows. Bring your arms back in to finish the move.

94 Hanging knee raise

TARGET Lower abs

DIFFICULTY RATING ●●●○○

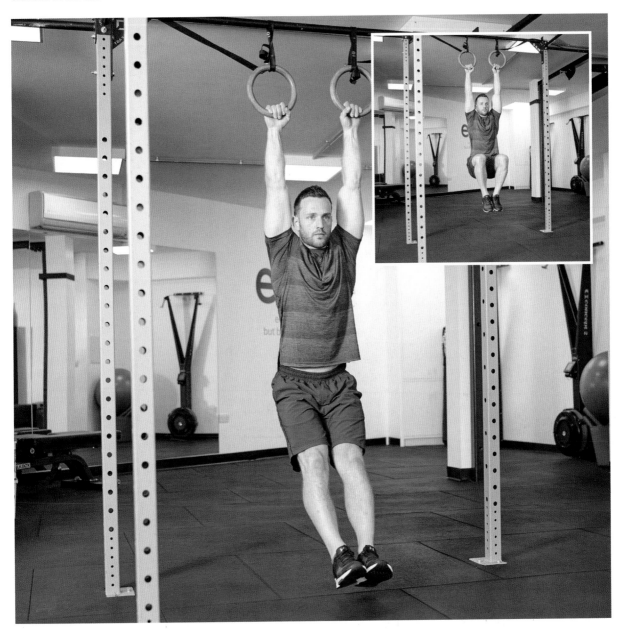

WHY As well as targeting your abs, this move works your grip, forcing you to stabilise yourself in the hang position while the rings move slightly.

HOW Hang from the rings. Bend your knees and use your lower abs to raise your legs until your thighs are parallel to the floor. Lower slowly back to the start.

95 Hanging leg raise

TARGET Lower abs

DIFFICULTY RATING ●●●○○

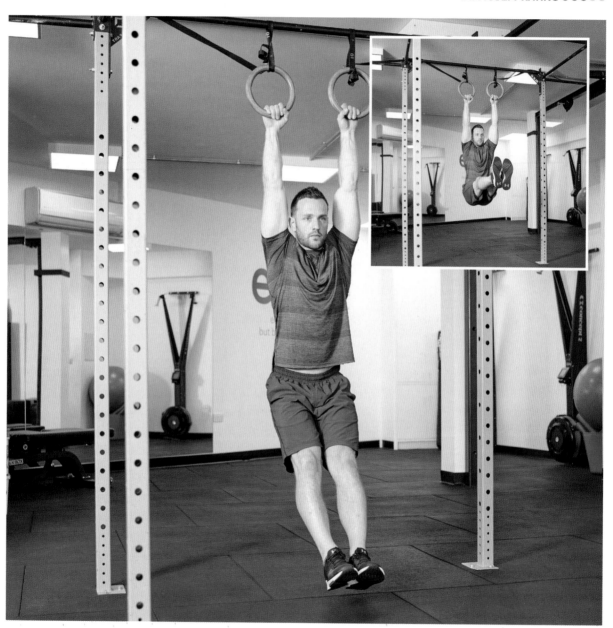

WHY Because it's tougher on the abs than the knee raise, you're more likely to hit failure on this move before your grip goes. For the ultimate challenge, go to failure on this and then do a few more reps of knee raises.

HOW Hang from the rings. Use your lower abs to raise your legs until your thighs are parallel to the floor. Lower slowly back to the start.

96 Inverted row

TARGET Back, biceps, abs and core

DIFFICULTY RATING ●●●○○

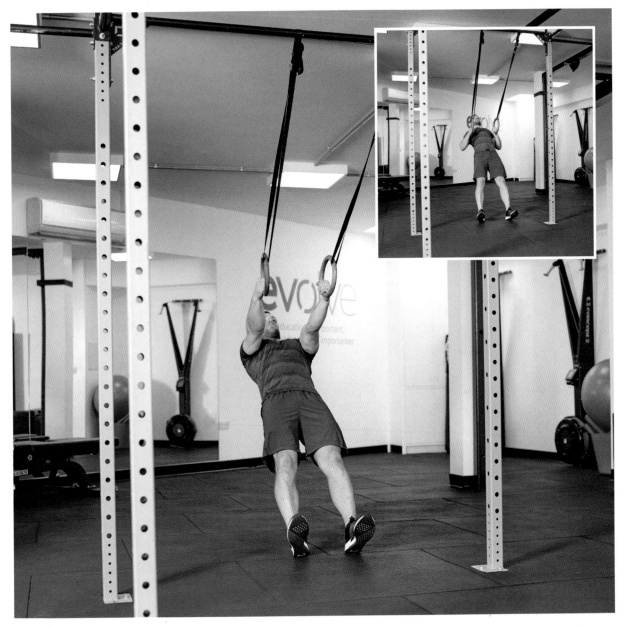

WHY As well as working your abs, this move will engage your shoulders and keep them healthy, while allowing your wrists to rotate naturally to reduce strain on your elbows.

HOW Hold the rings and lean back, keeping your body in a straight line. Focus on pulling your elbows behind you as you pull up to the rings. Lower back to the start under control.

97 L-sit

TARGET Abs and core

DIFFICULTY RATING ●●●○○

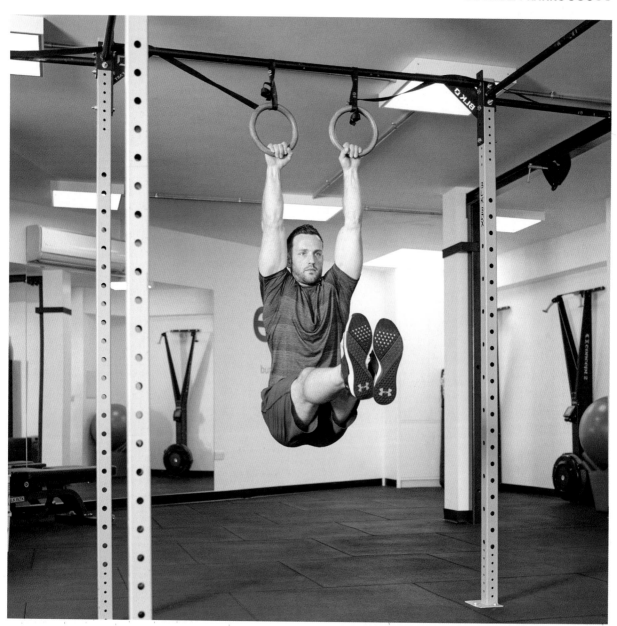

WHY This isometric move will build your functional abs strength. If it's too hard to start with, do it with your legs tucked. You can also do this from the hang position, but it's tougher.

HOW Hang from the rings. Bring your legs up until they're parallel to the floor, brace your abs and hold. Tucking forwards slightly will help with your balance.

98 Plank

TARGET Abs and core

DIFFICULTY RATING ●●●○○

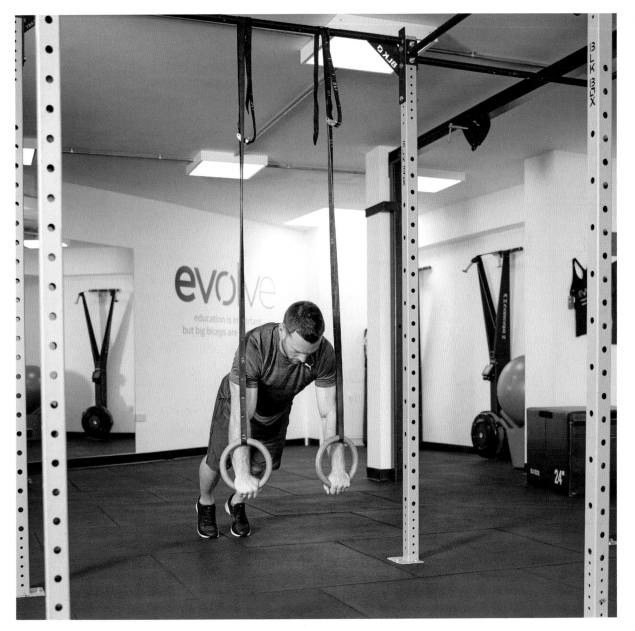

WHY If you can do more than two minutes of the regular plank, it's time to add instability. This move will work every part of your body but especially your core, which it'll put in overdrive.

HOW Hold the rings with your feet on the floor, leaning forward into the top position of a press-up. Brace your abs and glutes so that your body's straight, and hold.

99 Press-up

TARGET Chest, triceps, abs and core

DIFFICULTY RATING ●●●○○

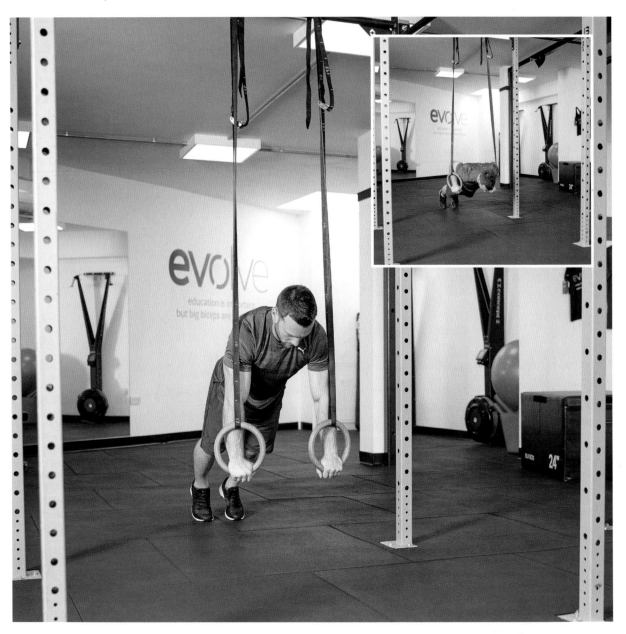

WHY It's much harder than the regular version, though keeping the rings close will help. The ring press-up will also put extra emphasis on your abs, working your core from all directions.

HOW Grasp the rings, lean forwards and lower until their edges touch your armpits, then press up. As you improve, lower the rings (or put your feet on a box) until you're closer to the angle of a standard press-up.

100 **Roll-out**

TARGET Abs and core

DIFFICULTY RATING ●●●○○

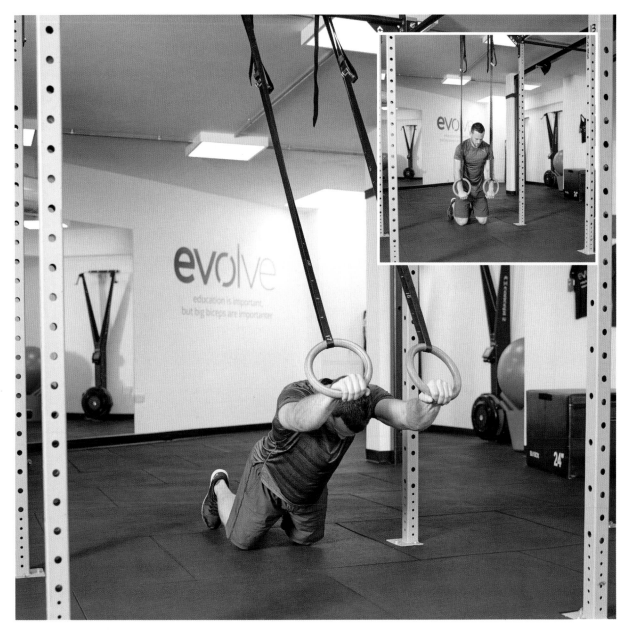

WHY Slightly tougher than the kneeling abs roll-out (see p57), this move lets you adjust the difficulty by moving the rings up or down. The closer you get to the floor, the harder it gets. It's a killer for your upper abs.

HOW Kneel holding the rings at waist height. Lean forwards, keeping your body in a straight line, and allow your arms to rise so they finish above your head. Brace your abs and pull the rings down to return to the start position.

101 Top position hold

TARGET Abs and core

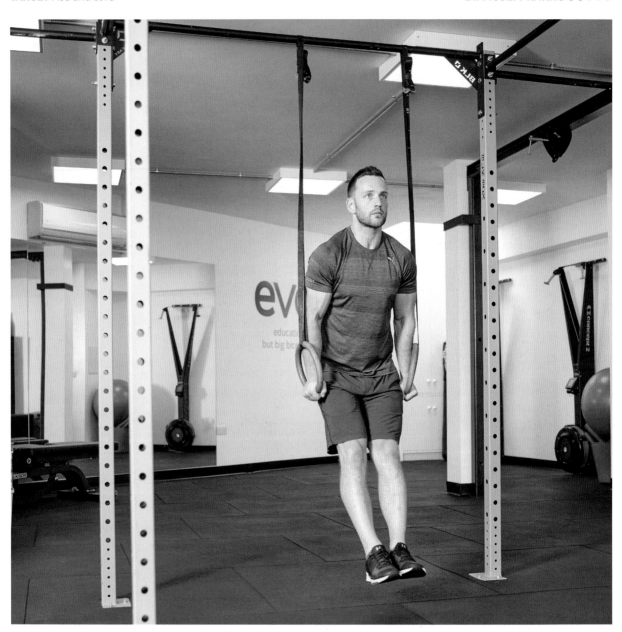

WHY Learning to stay stable and create tension helps you deal with the instability of the rings. Mastering this move will teach you to create locked-out strength in more advanced positions.

HOW Jump into the top position of a dip – elbows locked, rings close to your body. Hold for a second, then turn your hands outwards to feel the extra tension. Turn back in and repeat for as long as you can.

Mind, Body & Soul

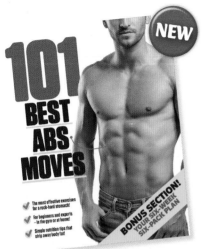

101 BEST ABS MOVES

NEW

- The most effective exercises for a rock-hard stomach!
- For beginners and experts – in the gym or at home!
- Simple nutrition tips that strip away body fat!

BONUS SECTION! YOUR SIX-WEEK SIX-PACK PLAN

When it comes to looking good, few can deny that a washboard six-pack of toned abs looks so much better than a flabby belly. The Complete Guide to Abs explains the simple steps you can take to sculpt your six-pack through a combination of regular exercise and healthy eating. You can also benefit from overall improved health and fitness as part of this straightforward programme.

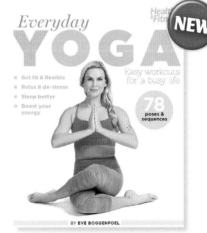

Everyday **YOGA**

Health & Fitness

NEW

Easy workouts for a busy life

- Get fit & flexible
- Relax & de-stress
- Sleep better
- Boost your energy

78 poses & sequences

BY EVE BOGGENPOEL

Until you've experienced it for yourself it's hard to really understand the difference a regular yoga practice can make to your life. People speak of improved flexibility, increased strength, better balance and greater stamina, but the benefits go far beyond the physical. Along with better sleep, deeper relaxation and greater focus you can get a feeling of purpose that is hard to beat.

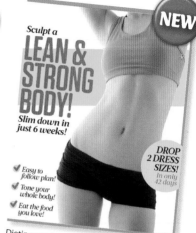

Sculpt a **LEAN & STRONG BODY!**

NEW

Slim down in just 6 weeks!

- Easy to follow plan!
- Tone your whole body!
- Eat the food you love!

DROP 2 DRESS SIZES! *In only 42 days*

Dieting can be tough and it's easy to fall off the wagon before you reach your goal - which is why Sculpt a Lean and Strong Body! helps you complete the journey from flabby couch potato to a lean and athletic physique through a simple exercise plan, a generous dietary programme and easily accomplished objectives.

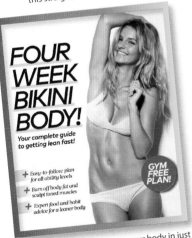

FOUR WEEK BIKINI BODY!

Your complete guide to getting lean fast!

GYM FREE PLAN!

- Easy-to-follow plan for all ability levels
- Burn off body fat and sculpt toned muscles
- Expert food and habit advice for a leaner body

Complete guide to toning up your body in just four weeks. Following a simple step-by-step programme, you'll burn more fat and develop lean, defined muscles. Plus, learn good habits that will make you healthier for life.

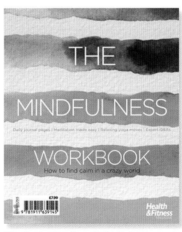

THE MINDFULNESS WORKBOOK

Daily journal pages | Meditation made easy | Relaxing yoga moves | Expert Q&As

How to find calm in a crazy world

Health & Fitness

If you're not exactly sure what being mindful involves, this is the place to start. Here you'll learn the history and main concepts of mindfulness, and get an idea of how your life might look after you learn to live more fully in the moment. Discover the ways mindfulness is used by its many advocates - from celebrities to professors - and learn how it can benefit you too.

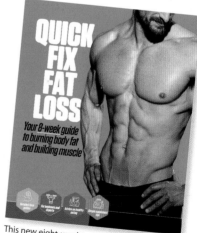

QUICK FIX FAT LOSS

Your 8-week guide to burning body fat and building muscle

This new eight-week training and eating plan that will help you shift body fat fast and allow you to build the body you've always wanted.

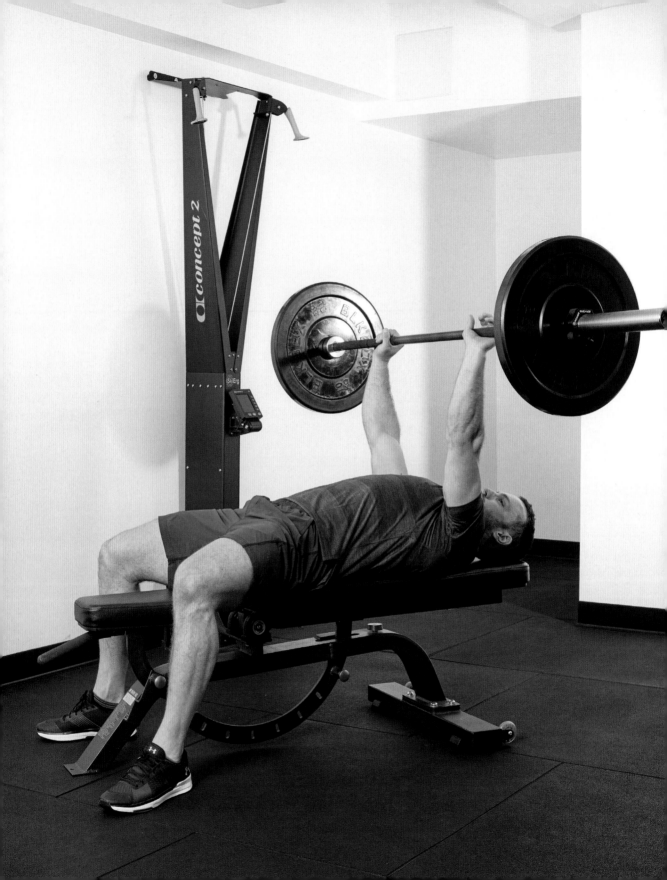

SIX-PACK IN SIX WEEKS

WEEK 1
WORKOUT 1

Get your six-week plan off to a strong start with this fun and challenging six-move session

You might be wondering why your six-week six-pack plan start with a squat – a move that primarily challenges your lower body. The reason is pretty simple. Big compound moves such as squats, which work multiple muscles groups simultaneously, are useful for a couple of reasons.

First, they'll help you burn calories, which means they'll reduce your body fat levels so that you can actually see the abs you're sculpting. Second, they are effective at challenging your abs and core because you need to activate the stabilising muscles that support your spine. For that reason, every workout in this initial three-week section of the plan starts with a superset

(two exercises performed back to back without rest, marked 1A and 1B) of big compound exercises – in this instance the squat and overhead press.

The remaining four exercises all work your abdominal muscles more directly but they do so in different ways. One of the exercises is designed to challenge your upper abs, one of them works your lower abs and another will test your side abs. Each workout in this three-week section ends with a static hold, which develops your core strength.

Make sure you stick to the set, rep and rest instructions to get the most out of the plan. And select a weight that allows you to just about complete the final move of the final set.

1A Barbell squat

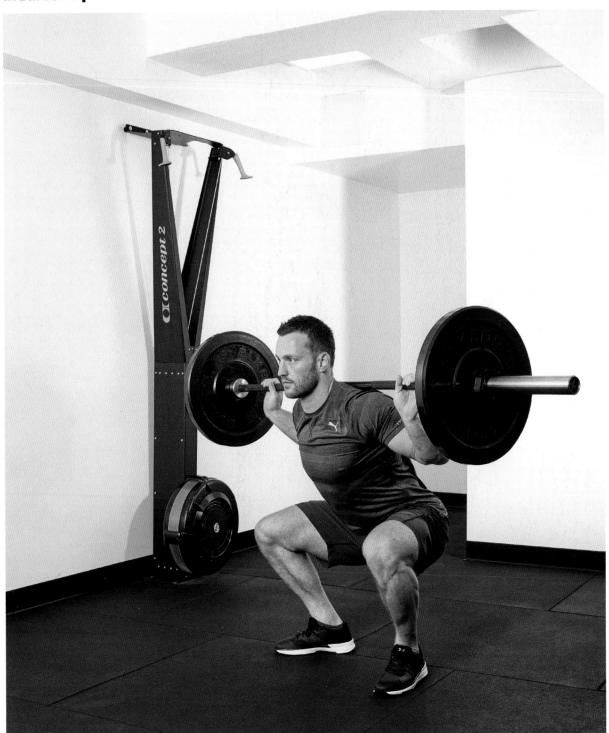

SETS 2 **REPS** 12-15 **REST** 0sec

FORM p62

1B Barbell overhead press

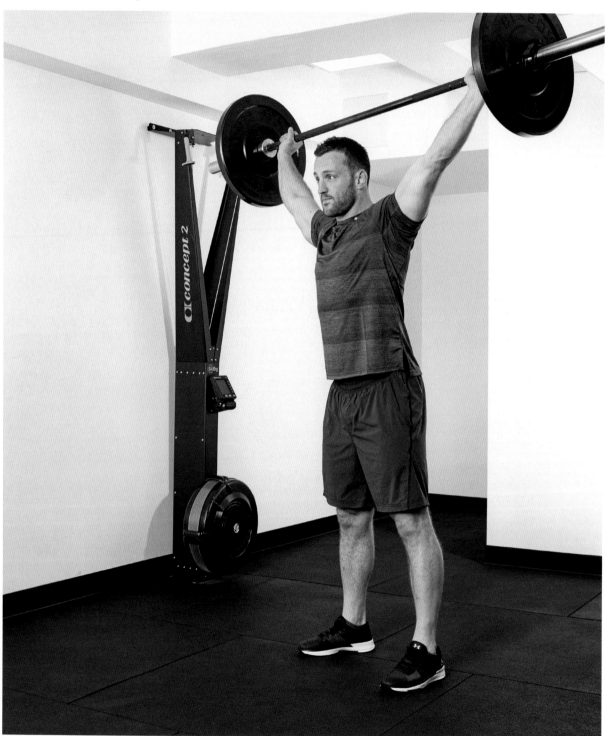

SETS 2 **REPS** 12-15 **REST** 60sec

FORM p59

2 Crunch

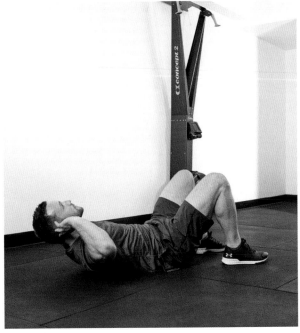

SETS 2 REPS 12-15 REST 60sec   FORM p13

3 Leg raise

SETS 2 REPS 12-15 REST 60sec   FORM p19

4 Russian twist

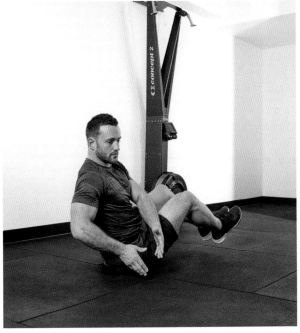

SETS 2 REPS 12-15 REST 60sec   FORM p27

5 Plank

SETS 2 TIME 30sec REST 60sec   FORM p22

WEEK 1 WORKOUT 2

The second session this week focuses on your upper body to build a lean, muscular physique

This workout follows the same pattern as the week's first session but uses different exercises to challenge different muscle groups. The superset at the start of the workout, the bench press and the bent-over row, is a classic combo for building your upper body.

When the bench press gets heavy it requires you to recruit your abs because you need a stable base from which you can press the weight. The bent-over row places a different demand on your core because you have to keep your torso fixed and stable as you raise and lower the bar. These two moves have been put together because they work antagonistic muscle groups (ones on opposite sides of your body), an approach that will give you balanced muscle development. If you just did the bench press and neglected your back muscles your shoulders would start to hunch forwards and you'd compromise your posture.

The final four exercises in this workout are all abs moves. The crunch reach is an excellent way of hitting your upper abs, the dish hold will work your upper and lower abs simultaneously and the heel touch is a great innovative move for targeting your side abs. The workout finishes with a side plank – a demanding static hold that places more emphasis on those side abs.

1A Barbell bench press

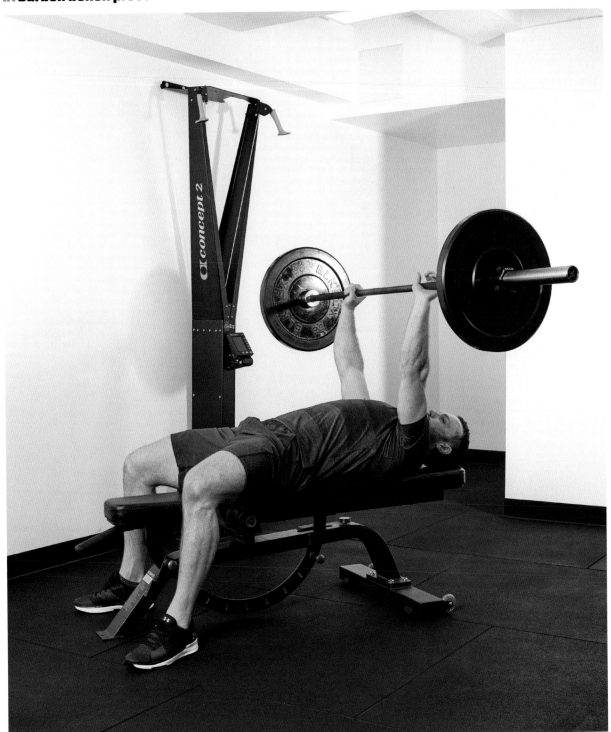

SETS 2 **REPS** 12–15 **REST** 0sec

FORM p52

1B Barbell bent-over row

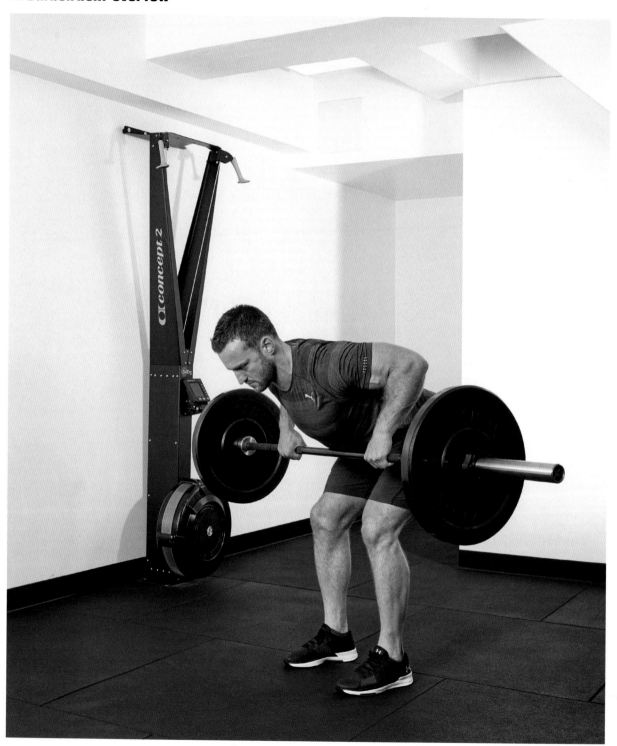

SETS 2 **REPS** 12–15 **REST** 60sec

FORM p53

2 Crunch reach

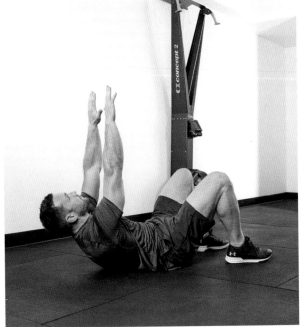

SETS 2 REPS 12-15 REST 60sec   FORM p14

3 Dish hold

SETS 2 REPS 12-15 REST 60sec   FORM p16

4 Heel touch

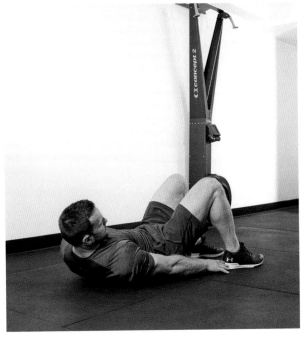

SETS 2 REPS 12-15 REST 60sec   FORM p17

5 Side plank

SETS 1 each side TIME 30sec REST 60sec   FORM p29

WEEK 1 WORKOUT 3

The final session of the week involves the king of lifts and some quirky abs exercises

This is the week's final session, so we want you to really push yourself and get the most you can out of the workout. Remember - the results you achieve will be directly proportionate to the effort you put into each session. That means really concentrating on every rep and thinking about the body part that you're trying to work.

The superset at the beginning of the workout is a deadlift followed by an overhead squat. These are both tough and technical exercises, so you really need to concentrate on your form to do them properly. The deadlift is arguably the best all-round exercise you can do. It works virtually every muscle group in your body and is the move that allows you to lift the most weight. The overhead squat is very useful for anyone who wants to build

a six-pack because it requires a huge amount of core strength to keep your torso stable as you lower with a barbell held above your head.

The abs moves in this workout will test your midsection in a variety of ways. The garhammar raise is one of the most effective exercises you can do for your hard-to-hit lower abs. It's deceptively difficult too – the movement may be small but it places a big demand on your muscles because it isolates the lower abs when it is done correctly. The plank touch at the end of the workout is an unusual and effective way to end your workout and your training week.

In the following two weeks the exercise selection remains the same but the variables – such as sets, reps and rest – will change.

1A Barbell deadlift

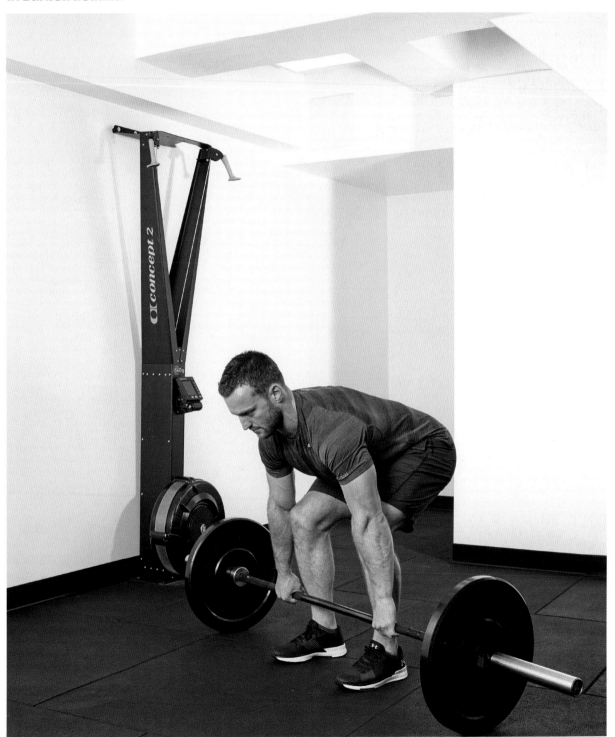

SETS 2 **REPS** 12-15 **REST** 0sec

FORM p54

1B Barbell overhead squat

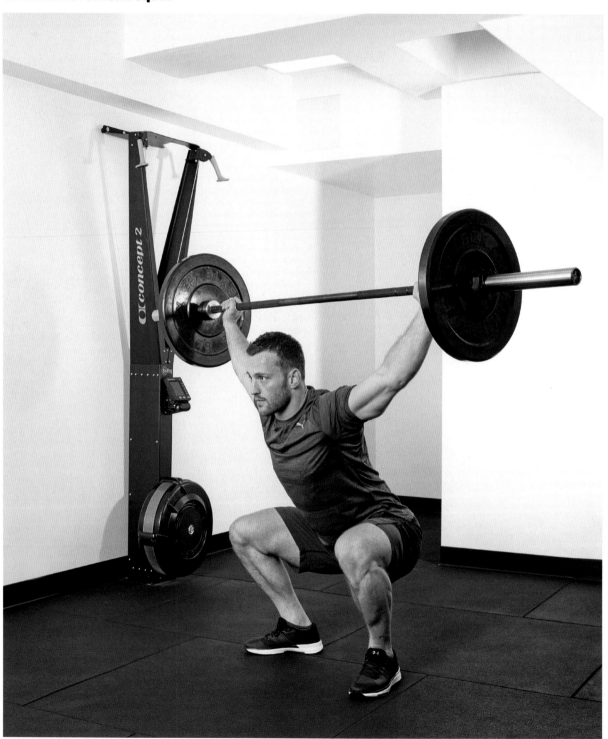

SETS 2 **REPS** 12-15 **REST** 60sec

FORM p60

2 Hanging knee raise

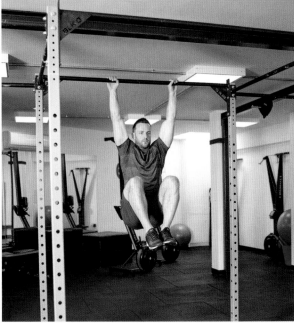

SETS 2 **REPS** 12-15 **REST** 60sec   **FORM** p110

3 Garhammer raise

SETS 2 **REPS** 12-15 **REST** 60sec   **FORM** p108

4 Bicycle

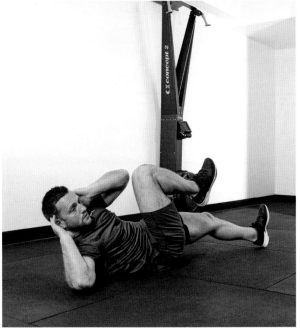

SETS 2 **REPS** 12-15 **REST** 60sec   **FORM** p12

5 Plank touch

SETS 2 **TIME** 30sec **REST** 60sec   **FORM** p24

WEEK 2

Workout 1

EXERCISE	SETS	REPS/TIME	REST
1A Barbell squat	3	10	0sec
1B Barbell overhead press	3	10	60sec
2 Crunch	3	10	60sec
3 Leg raise	3	10	60sec
4 Russian twist	3	10	60sec
5 Plank	3	40sec	60sec

Workout 2

EXERCISE	SETS	REPS/TIME	REST
1A Barbell bench press	3	10	0sec
1B Barbell bent-over row	3	10	60sec
2 Crunch reach	3	10	60sec
3 Dish hold	3	10	60sec
4 Heel touch	3	10	60sec
5 Side plank	3	40sec	60sec

Workout 3

EXERCISE	SETS	REPS/TIME	REST
1A Barbell deadlift	3	10	0sec
1B Barbell overhead squat	3	10	60sec
2 Hanging knee raise	3	10	60sec
3 Garhammer raise	3	10	60sec
4 Bicycle	3	10	60sec
5 Plank touch	3	40sec	60sec

WEEK 3

Workout 1

EXERCISE	SETS	REPS/TIME	REST
1A Barbell squat	3	12	0sec
1B Barbell overhead press	3	12	60sec
2 Crunch	3	12	60sec
3 Leg raise	3	12	60sec
4 Russian twist	3	12	60sec
5 Plank	3	50sec	60sec

Workout 2

EXERCISE	SETS	REPS/TIME	REST
1A Barbell bench press	3	12	0sec
1B Barbell bent-over row	3	12	60sec
2 Crunch reach	3	12	60sec
3 Dish hold	3	12	60sec
4 Heel touch	3	12	60sec
5 Side plank	3	50sec	60sec

Workout 3

EXERCISE	SETS	REPS/TIME	REST
1A Barbell deadlift	3	12	0sec
1B Barbell overhead squat	3	12	60sec
2 Hanging knee raise	3	12	60sec
3 Garhammer raise	3	12	60sec
4 Bicycle	3	12	60sec
5 Plank touch	3	50sec	60sec

WEEK 4 WORKOUT 1

Get the week off to a swinging start by picking up a kettlebell and building explosive strength

You're now halfway through your six-week plan and you should be seeing some solid results. The aim of the first three weeks was to combine some big compound strength moves, such as squats and deadlifts, with a balanced selection of abs-focused exercises that would hit your six-pack from different angles. The second half of the programme take a bit of a twist. Each workout in each week is devoted to one item of kit.

The first workout of the week features kettlebells, which are versatile pieces of functional training kit that get you moving fluidly. The unstable nature of the exercises requires your body to recruit its deep-lying core muscles as well as the muscles closer to the surface that make up your six-pack.

The workout begins with the kettlebell snatch. The key with this move is to concentrate on a hip snap to generate the power that will raise the bell above your head. In other word it's your hips, not your arms and shoulders, that should be doing the work. The second exercise - rolling thunder - is a fun way of working your abs and it looks pretty cool too.

The next exercise is a real test of side abs strength and shoulder stability, so start light and add weight as you get more familiar with the exercise. The halo, angel press and plank drag all offer challenging but engaging ways to train your abs. You will be tired at the end of this tough workout but one thing's for sure – you won't be bored.

1 Snatch

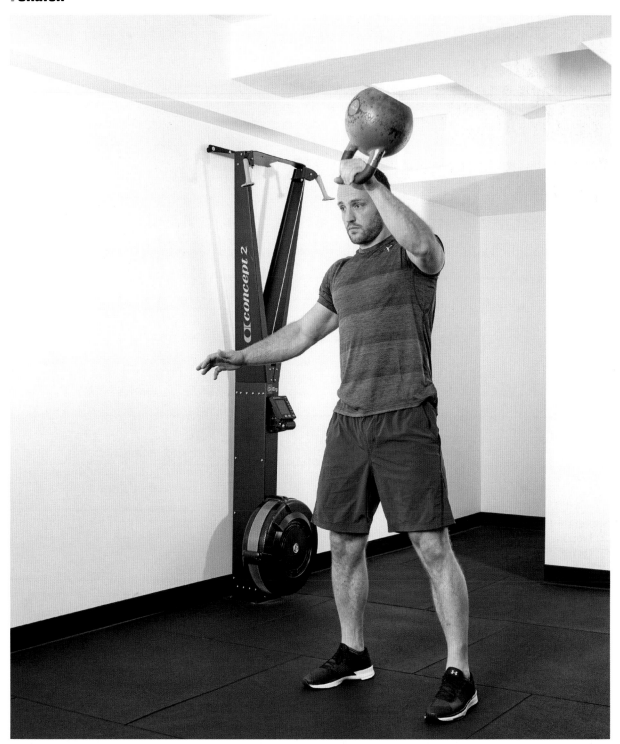

SETS 2 **REPS** 12-15 **REST** 60sec

FORM p75

2 Rolling thunder

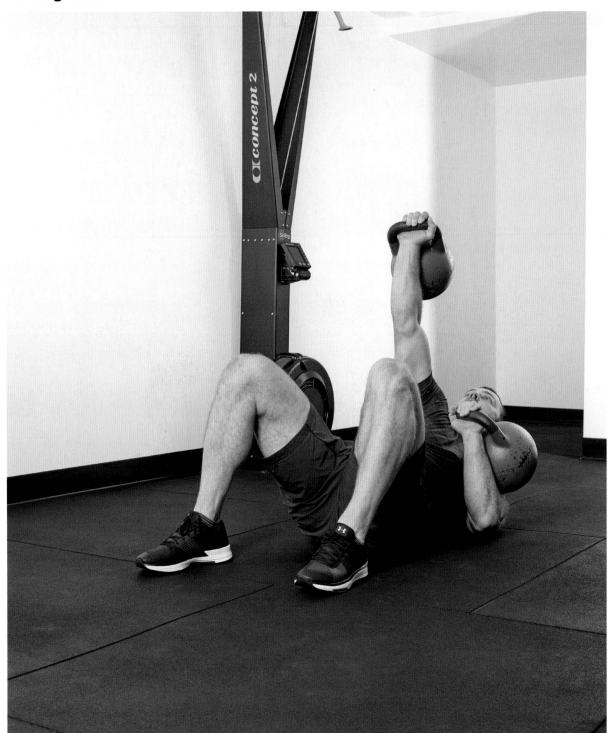

SETS 2 **REPS** 12–15 **REST** 60sec

FORM p72

3 Windmill

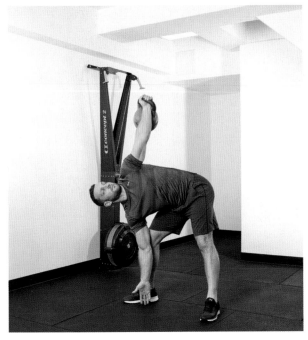

SETS 2 REPS 10 each side REST 60sec   FORM p77

4 Halo

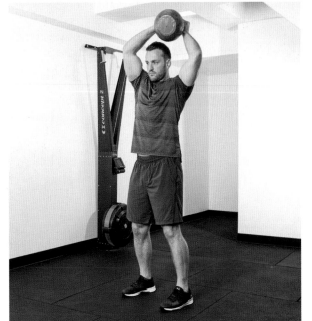

SETS 2 REPS 12-15 REST 60sec   FORM p69

5 Angel press

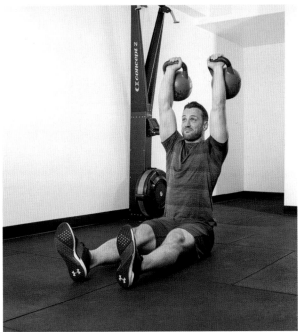
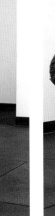

SETS 2 REPS 6-8 REST 60sec   FORM p66

6 Plank pass

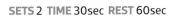

SETS 2 TIME 30sec REST 60sec   FORM p70

WEEK 4 WORKOUT 2

It's time to chuck your weight around by using a medicine ball to sculpt a six-pack

The second workout this week follows the same format as the first. All you need is one item of kit and, in this instance, that item is a medicine ball.

Medicine balls are a lot of fun to use because you can chuck them around and this workout includes plenty of throwing exercises. The reason throws are so useful is that they are explosive exercises you can do at maximum intensity yet they present minimal injury risk. Other explosive exercises, such as Olympic lifting exercises performed with a bar, offer the same kind of benefits but take a lot longer to master and also increase your risk of injury.

In the first exercise of this session you throw the ball overhead so you're going from low to high. In the second move – forming a superset with the first – you're going from high to low but you've also got to control the deceleration. Changing position in this way requires you to coordinate your upper and lower body, and that means you need a strong and stable core to execute the move under control. The act of straightening up with your arms above your head and then bringing your torso forwards and your arms down in front of you mimics the crunch movement but does it in a functional way.

Medicine balls can also be used to make exercises more unstable. When you perform a press-up with one hand on the ball your abs and core have to work harder than they would do in a conventional press-up to stabilise your body and prevent you from losing your balance. The same concept applies when you perform a plank with your hands on the medicine ball. So, attack the workout – and make sure you enjoy it!

1A Overhead throw

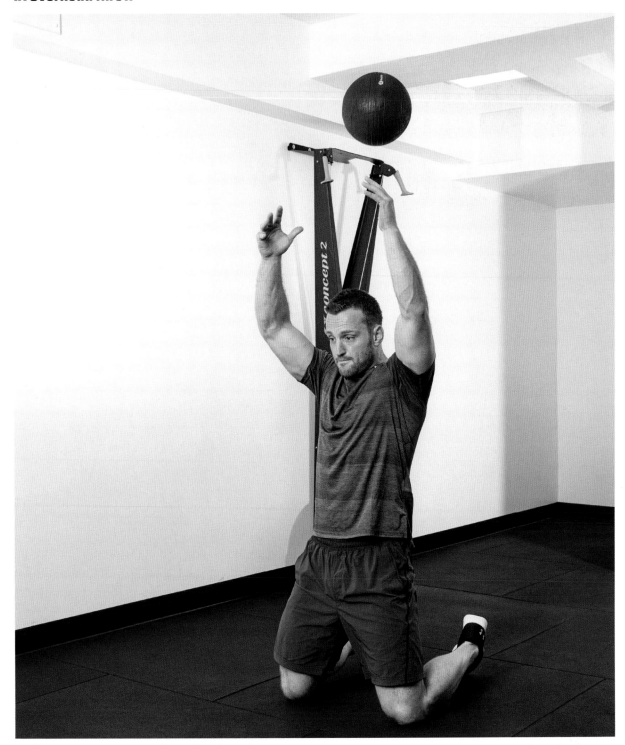

1B Sledgehammer

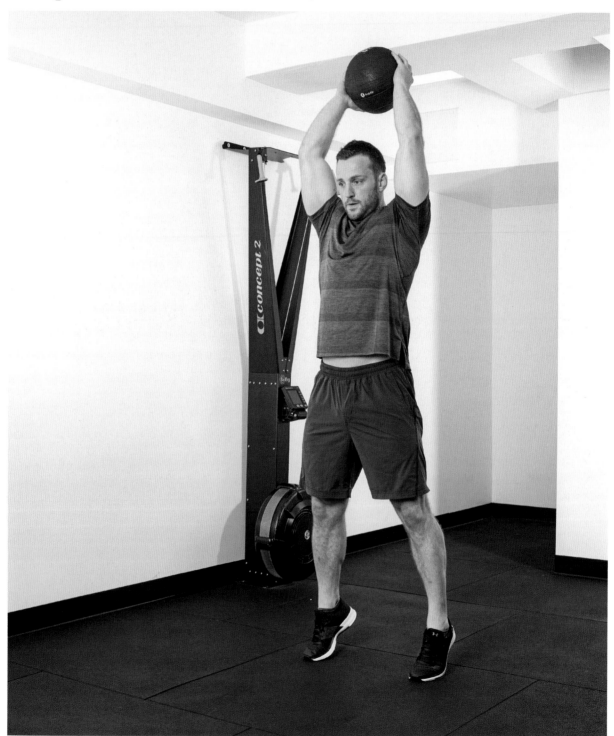

SETS 2 **REPS** 12–15 **REST** 60sec

FORM p90

2 Passing press-up

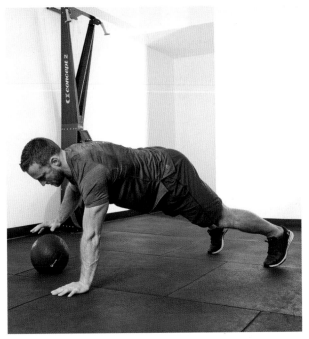

SETS 2 **REPS** 12-15 **REST** 60sec   **FORM** p85

3 Lying knee raise

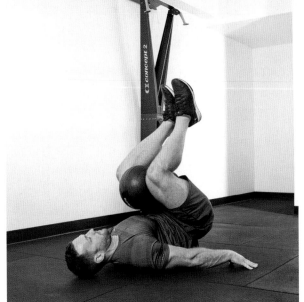

SETS 2 **REPS** 12-15 **REST** 60sec   **FORM** p82

4 Side throw

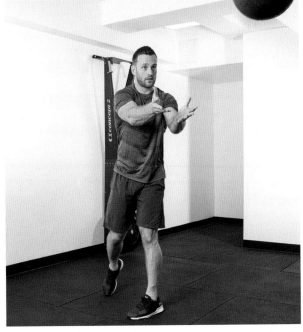

SETS 2 **REPS** 12-15 **REST** 60sec   **FORM** p91

5 Plank

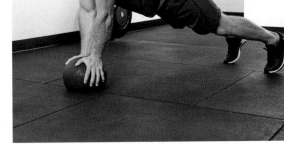

SETS 2 **TIME** 30sec **REST** 60sec   **FORM** p86

WEEK 4 WORKOUT 3

The final workout of the week uses rings to target better core strength and stability

Rings and other suspension training devices such as TRX have become increasingly popular in recent years and with good reason. They're accessible, versatile bits of kit and they are excellent at training your abs and core. The reason they are so good at building abs strength is that they make every exercise unstable. And the more unstable an exercise is, the harder your abs and core have to work to control your body position.

This session starts with an exercise designed to activate your muscles and get your mind used to the unstable nature of the rings. The next two moves, which should be done as a superset (back to back without rest), are the rings equivalents of the bench press and bent-over row superset that you did with a barbell in weeks 1-3. The

ring press-up will require a lot of strength and core control, as well as shoulder stability. The inverted row will ensure that your muscle development is balanced because it works the back of your body. One tip we'd give you is to tense your glutes throughout the set – that will send the right signal to your spinal stabilisers and help you to maintain a good position.

The ring roll-out is one of the most effective abs exercises you can do. It's also arguably easier to perform than the barbell version because you can set the rings at a height that suits your ability. The lower the rings, the harder the exercise. Even the humble plank is brought to life when using a set of rings. If you're not shaking by the end of your set, you have some impressive core control.

1 Top position hold

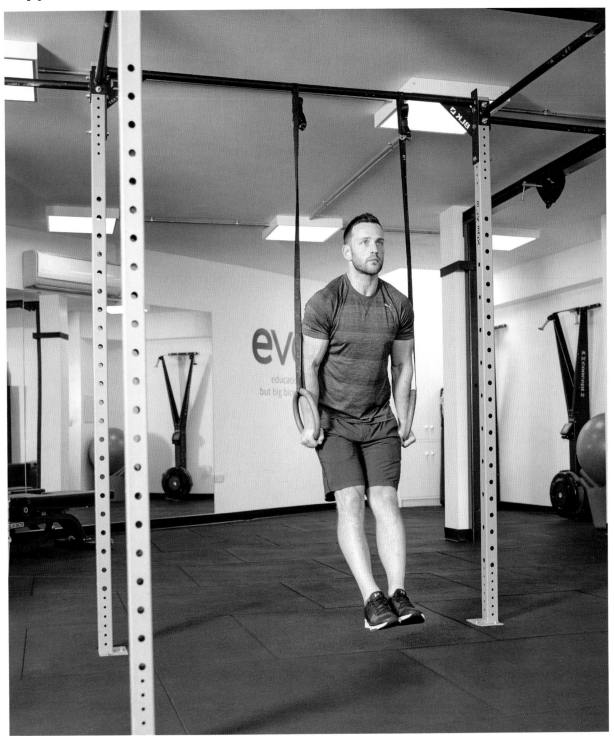

SETS 2 **TIME** 20sec **REST** 60sec

FORM p126

2A Press-up

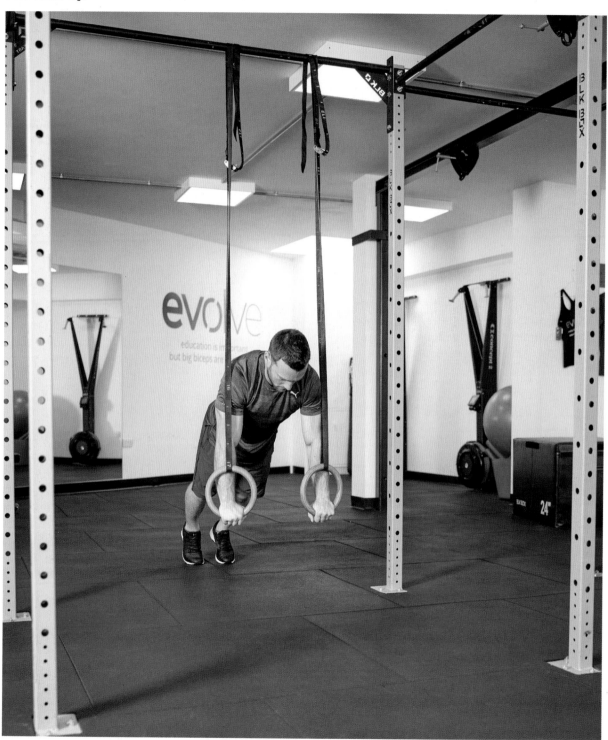

SETS 2 **REPS** 8–10 **REST** 0sec

FORM p124

2B Inverted row

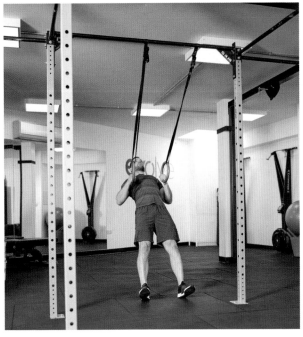

SETS 2 REPS 8-10 REST 60sec   FORM p121

3 Hanging knee raise

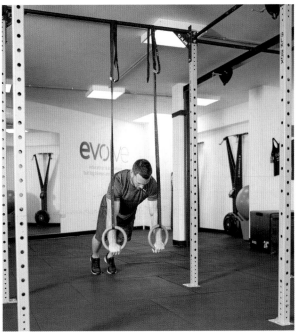

SETS 2 REPS 12-15 REST 60sec   FORM p119

4 Roll-out

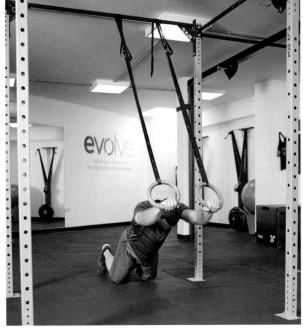

SETS 2 REPS 12-15 REST 60sec   FORM p125

5 Plank

SETS 2 TIME 20sec REST 60sec   FORM p123

WEEK 5

Workout 1

EXERCISE	SETS	REPS/TIME	REST
1 Snatch	3	10	60sec
2 Rolling thunder	3	10	60sec
3 Windmill	3	10	60sec
4 Halo	3	10	60sec
5 Angel press	3	8-10	60sec
6 Plank pass	3	30sec	60sec

Workout 2

EXERCISE	SETS	REPS/TIME	REST
1A Overhead throw	3	10	0sec
1B Sledgehammer	3	10	60sec
2 Passing press-up	3	10	60sec
3 Lying knee raise	3	10	60sec
4 Side throw	3	10	60sec
5 Plank	3	30sec	60sec

Workout 3

EXERCISE	SETS	REPS/TIME	REST
1 Top position hold	3	10	60sec
2A Press-up	3	10	0sec
2B Inverted row	3	10	60sec
3 Hanging knee raise	3	10	60sec
4 Roll-out	3	10	60sec
5 Plank	3	30sec	60sec

WEEK 6

Workout 1

EXERCISE	SETS	REPS/TIME	REST
1 Snatch	3	12	60sec
2 Rolling thunder	3	12	60sec
3 Windmill	3	12	60sec
4 Halo	3	12	60sec
5 Angel press	3	10-12	60sec
6 Plank pass	3	40sec	60sec

Workout 2

EXERCISE	SETS	REPS/TIME	REST
1A Overhead throw	3	12	0sec
1B Sledgehammer	3	12	60sec
2 Passing press-up	3	12	60sec
3 Lying knee raise	3	12	60sec
4 Side throw	3	12	60sec
5 Plank	3	40sec	60sec

Workout 3

EXERCISE	SETS	REPS/TIME	REST
1 Top position hold	3	12	60sec
2A Press-up	3	12	0sec
2B Inverted row	3	12	60sec
3 Hanging knee raise	3	12	60sec
4 Roll-out	3	12	60sec
5 Plank	3	40sec	60sec

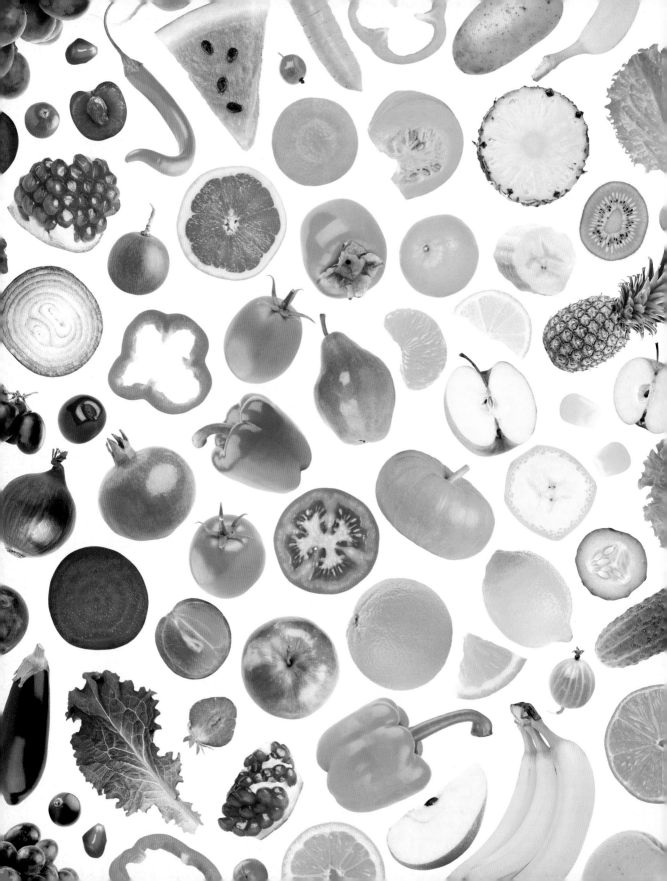

EAT
FOR
ABS

7 RULES OF EATING FOR A SIX-PACK

Follow these seven smart food strategies to transform your body

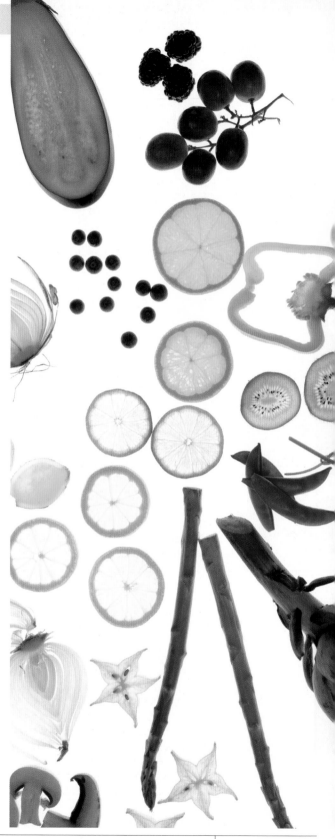

NEVER SKIP BREAKFAST

Breakfast is called the most important meal of the day with good reason. Your body has been deprived of energy and nutrients for the eight hours you've been asleep, so starting your day with smart food choices is crucial – it will help your body burn fat throughout the day and keep blood sugar levels stable so that hunger is kept at bay and you're not tempted to eat high-sugar and high-fat foods.

Eating the right foods for breakfast – which means high-protein foods such as eggs, smoked salmon, good-quality sausages and even steak, alongside fibre-rich foods like mushrooms, tomatoes, avocado and greens – will also improve your focus, motivation and willpower, and you need all three to ensure you stick to your both your training programme and your new healthy-eating diet plan. And if you think skipping breakfast is a shortcut to the fat loss you need in order to display your six-pack to full effect, think again: research proves people who don't eat brekkie consume more total calories over the course of the entire day than those who do.

KEEP IT NATURAL

All the food you put in your shopping basket from now on should be in as close to its natural form as possible. That means stocking your fridge with

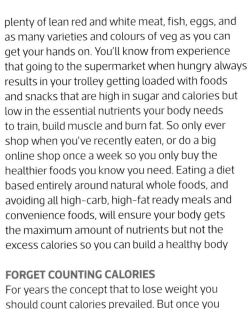
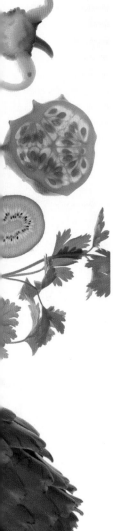

plenty of lean red and white meat, fish, eggs, and as many varieties and colours of veg as you can get your hands on. You'll know from experience that going to the supermarket when hungry always results in your trolley getting loaded with foods and snacks that are high in sugar and calories but low in the essential nutrients your body needs to train, build muscle and burn fat. So only ever shop when you've recently eaten, or do a big online shop once a week so you only buy the healthier foods you know you need. Eating a diet based entirely around natural whole foods, and avoiding all high-carb, high-fat ready meals and convenience foods, will ensure your body gets the maximum amount of nutrients but not the excess calories so you can build a healthy body

FORGET COUNTING CALORIES

For years the concept that to lose weight you should count calories prevailed. But once you realise that not all calories are created equal, you can't help but see the flaw in this system. Still need convincing? What's the better option if you want to burn fat: 150 calories from two boiled eggs (containing quality protein and fat) or 150 calories from a muffin (all carbs, mainly sugar)? It's not tricky – so don't get caught up in this calorie-counting confusion. Your body is going to need plenty of high-quality protein and fats to support your exercise efforts and aid recovery so you can keep moving towards your goal. If you're unsure how this works in practice, just follow the next four rules and you won't go too far wrong.

GET MORE PROTEIN

If you don't eat enough good-quality protein – think meat, fish and eggs – then don't be surprised if you fail to make the progress you want as quickly as you'd like. The reason is simple. When you work out you cause small, microscopic tears in your muscles so you need to eat more protein – which is made up of amino acids, which are the building blocks of muscle – so you body has the right nutrients needed to repair this damage and rebuild your muscles bigger and stronger. As well as helping your build your six-pack, this will also help you reveal it because muscle is active tissue – which means the more muscle you have, the more calories your body will burn, even at rest.

Aim for a fist-sized serving of protein for every meal, and spend a little more money if you can to buy organic and grass-fed produce because it contains more vitamins, minerals and omega 3 fatty acids, which will also boost the fat burn.

EAT MORE VEG

If you struggle to get your five-a-day then you need to up your game because you need to have veg – and a wide variety of it – with every meal you eat. It's packed with the vitamins and minerals your body will be crying out for after training, as well as fibre to keep you feeling fuller for longer and stabilise your blood sugar levels so you won't be tempted by sweet snacks.

If you really dislike vegetables there are some simple ways to make them more palatable. Try adding butter once you've plated up to improve flavour and help vitamin absorption, or cook them with garlic, chilli or any other herbs and spices you like to add some flavour.

REMEMBER FAT IS YOUR FRIEND

Fat in food was vilified for decades for causing health problems ranging from obesity to heart disease. But the research behind these claims has been largely discredited and the importance of fats to a healthy diet – especially with regards to better hormone function, which will help you burn body fat – are now widely recognised. The exception is trans fats, which are unnatural, man-made fats found in fast food and heavily processed sweets and snacks. This type of fat is not found in natural food so your body doesn't know how to deal with it, and eating it can cause all kinds of unpleasant health problems.

STOP DRINKING SUGAR

One of the easiest ways to improve your diet is to stop drinking so many calories, especially the nutrient-free calories found in fizzy drinks and processed fruit juices. These drinks have little to no nutritional value and should be completely avoided if you care about losing your belly – and about your overall health for that matter. Ideally, you should drink only three things: water (aim for at least two litres per day, and even more on days you work out); coffee (black is best); and tea (green tea is great, builder's tea with four sugars is bad).

BUILD HEALTHY HABITS

Implement these lifestyle routines to help blast away your belly and reveal your six-pack

WAKE UP WITH WATER

As soon as you get up – even before you go to the loo – down a pint of cold water. You awake in a dehydrated state and it's crucial to replace the water you've lost overnight (through sweating and simply breathing) as quickly as you can. Dehydration is a leading cause of poor mental and physical performance, both of which you want to avoid as much as possible to stay focused and motivated for your training goals. Always carry a big bottle of water around with you and sip from it constantly throughout the day to keep hydrated at all times.

EAT AT THE SAME TIMES

You don't need to eat like clockwork but try to eat breakfast, lunch and dinner at roughly the same times each day. This will soon establish a regular routine where you think nothing of finding the time to sit down and eat properly. Taking your time to eat can go a long way to maximising the nutritional impact of the wholesome food you're consuming, whereas eating in a rushed or stressed state won't. Eating at set times also removes the risk that you'll skip meals or go for long periods without eating anything, which more often than not results in cravings for high-sugar and high-fat snacks and convenience foods.

KEEP A FOOD DIARY

If you are really struggling to stay on top of your diet, start writing a food diary. You don't need to write down every single calorie you consume, or even the number of grams of protein you've eaten. A simple ballpark figure of what you ate and how much of it, as well as notes on how you feel – especially your energy and motivation levels – will give you a good steer on where you are going right or what you might be doing wrong, allowing you to make small and sensible changes to your nutritional approach and keep moving closer to finding the best dietary strategy for you.

BE CLEVER WITH CARBS

If you're trying to build muscle while burning fat, which you need to do to create an impressive six-pack, you need to be smart when selecting the carbs you eat. There's no need to eliminate all carbohydrates from your diet – that would be mean (carbs are delicious, after all) and unnecessary. But it's best to avoid all types of sugar, and limit consumption of fast-release carbs, like processed white bread, pasta and rice, all of which have been stripped of many of their nutrients and much of their fibre content. This means the energy from these carbs is digested, and so enter your bloodstream, quicker and cause a blood sugar spike, which leaves you craving food you don't really need.

To lose fat faster you want blood sugar levels that are as stable as possible. So your carbs should come from slow-release sources, like sweet potatoes and brown rice, as well as plenty of fibre-rich, nutrient-dense veg. Basically, you can't eat too many vegetables when you're working towards a fitness goal. The more the better.

DOUBLE DOWN AT DINNER

When making dinner, double the ingredients and make two portions so that you will have leftovers ready for tomorrow's lunch. This will not only save you time and money, it will also make it much easier for you to eat healthily and keep you on the path to a better body. If you can make the time, batch-cook two or three different meals at the weekend and keep them in the fridge or freezer, then simply reheat them throughout the week.